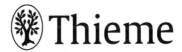

Auriculotherapy

Raphael Nogier, MD

President
Ecole Internationale Paul Nogier
Lyon, France

150 illustrations

Thieme
Stuttgart · New York

Library of Congress Cataloging-in-Publication Data

Nogier, Raphaël.
[Auriculothérapie, ou, L'acupuncture auriculaire 1er degré. English]
Auriculotherapy/Raphael Nogier;
[translator, Peter Beauclerk;
illustration of the ears, Cecile Begeron].
p.; cm.
Authorized and rev. translation of the French editions published and copyrighted 2006 by Sauramps Medical, Montpellier, France.
Includes bibliographical references.
ISBN 978-3-13-148001-9 (alk. paper)
1. Ear-Acupuncture. I. Nogier, Raphaël.
Auriculothérapie 2ème degré. English. II. Title.
[DNLM: 1. Acupuncture, Ear.
WB 369.5.E2 N777a 2008a]
RM184.N895513 2008
615.8'92–dc22

                     2008032143

© 2009 Georg Thieme Verlag,
Rüdigerstrasse 14, 70469 Stuttgart, Germany
http://www.thieme.de
Thieme New York, 333 Seventh Avenue,
New York, NY 10001, USA
http://www.thieme.com

Cover design: Thieme Publishing Group
Typesetting by Druckerei Sommer,
Feuchtwangen
Printed in Germany by Beltz Grafische Betriebe

ISBN: 978-3-13-148001-9

              5 6

Important note: Medicine is an ever-changing science undergoing continual development. Research and clinical experience are continually expanding our knowledge, in particular our knowledge of proper treatment and drug therapy. Insofar as this book mentions any dosage or application, readers may rest assured that the authors, editors, and publishers have made every effort to ensure that such references are in accordance with **the state of knowledge at the time of production of the book.**
Nevertheless, this does not involve, imply, or express any guarantee or responsibility on the part of the publishers in respect to any dosage instructions and forms of applications stated in the book. **Every user is requested to examine carefully** the manufacturers' leaflets accompanying each drug and to check, if necessary in consultation with a physician or specialist, whether the dosage schedules mentioned therein or the contraindications stated by the manufacturers differ from the statements made in the present book. Such examination is particularly important with drugs that are either rarely used or have been newly released on the market. Every dosage schedule or every form of application used is entirely at the user's own risk and responsibility. The authors and publishers request every user to report to the publishers any discrepancies or inaccuracies noticed. If errors in this work are found after publication, errata will be posted at www.thieme.com on the product description page.

Foreword

I met Raphael Nogier in 1978 when I was his interpreter for a series of auriculotherapy lectures in California. The following year we traveled together in China as participants in the first French–Chinese medical acupuncture exchange. Since then we have served together on WHO scientific committees to standardize acupuncture nomenclature, and we meet at international acupuncture congresses in various parts of the world. For three decades I have followed with admiration his contributions to the evolution of medical acupuncture, and was delighted when Thieme decided to publish an English edition of his recent synthesis of auriculotherapy.

Most practicing acupuncturists who consult this book will have already been exposed to the basic principles and practices of auriculotherapy, and possibly auriculomedicine. The text is directed at this audience. The author quickly reviews the background, theoretical foundations, and anatomy of auriculotherapy, and spends the first half of the book giving therapeutic guidelines for problems that commonly are successfully addressed with this technique. The table of contents serves as the constant reference as you scan for the illness you want to treat. Dr. Nogier has created an outline-plus-illustration format that enables practitioners to follow his logic and locate his suggested points with a minimum of words or confusion. I find this feature of the book very appealing, because translations of earlier French treatises on auriculotherapy and auriculomedicine tend to force the reader through a forest of phrases before finding what is sought … the treatment recommendation.

The disorders discussed in the first half of the book range from tobacco addiction to anxiety, and from sciatica to hemorrhoids … a wonderfully realistic and pragmatic collection. The second half of the book is more personalized. It covers more complex layers of anatomy and relationships among points, and leads to an outline-plus-illustration exploration of the phase theory, the vascular autonomic signal, and the Nogier frequencies. Appropriate to the complexity and elegance of the material, the disorders discussed in this final section of the book—such as fibromyalgia and depression—require more complex evaluation before treatment.

As a serious physician, observer, and teacher, Dr. Nogier has applied, clarified, and refined the discipline of auriculotherapy. During his decades of clinical practice, he has rigorously evaluated new applications of the technique and their scientific correlations. His practice of auriculotherapy has enabled him to study dietary allergies and their role in medical problems, and insights from his clinical experience in this field are included in the book.

You will find Raphael Nogier's *Auriculotherapy* a generous and practical companion that enhances your clinical appreciation of this discipline. He has brought his experience, pragmatism, and the humility that accompanies every good physician into this book, which magnifies the admirable work of his father and moves auriculotherapy one more step into the world of integrated medical practice.

Joseph M. Helms, M.D.
President, Helms Medical Institute, Berkeley, California
Founding President, American Academy of Medical Acupuncture

Introduction to Auriculotherapy

Paul Nogier was born 100 years ago in 1908. After a life passionately devoted to science and medicine, he bequeathed a most marvelous heritage both to the medical community and to society at large: auriculotherapy. This simple and effective technique is based on the reflexive properties inherent in the rich and complex innervation of the auricle of the ear. It provides physicians and appropriately trained paramedical professionals with a rapid and effective treatment modality for relieving the pain and functional problems associated with many medical complaints.

The birthplace of auriculotherapy is Lyon, and as a native of that city it is my pleasure to be able to introduce this technique, as presented in this book, to the English-speaking world. As the only one of Paul Nogier's sons to become a physician, I had the good fortune to work with him for many years. This gave me the opportunity to come to understand his thinking about auricular reflexotherapy as well as about medicine in general.

The fruit of many years of practice and teaching, this simple and straightforward book outlines the fundamental knowledge essential for understanding auriculotherapy. It is intended to enable those unfamiliar with the technique to start using it effectively in their practice, and for those already practicing it to further develop their skills.

I would like to thank Françoise Bourdiol for granting permission to publish the various drawings by her late husband René Bourdiol, MD, close collaborator and friend of Paul Nogier. My thanks also go to Joseph Helms for his considerate foreword, to Cécile Bergeron for her drawings, to Peter Beauclerk for the translation of the text, to Angelika Findgott and Thieme Publishers, and finally to Diana Bittner for her assistance in the book's preparation.

I dedicate this book to the following colleagues with whom I have worked closely in the past few years: Professor Pierre Magnin, who has guided me in my medical vocation, and Drs. Daniel Asis, Francis Baudet, Jorge Boucinhas, Bernard Bricot, Alain Coutté, Jean Goris, Rudolf Helling, Virginio Mariani, Michel Marignan, Simao, Yves Rouxeville, Anthony de Sousa, Paul de Susini, and Anne Marie Vester, Chantal Vulliez.

May this small work aid in the relief of those who suffer from pain and disease.

Raphael Nogier, MD

Table of Contents

Auriculotherapy in Medicine

The three factors determining health are:
- The way people live, which is culturally determined
- Hygiene
- Medicine, whose beneficial contribution is especially important during the perinatal period

Disorders are mainly caused by:
- The way people live—road traffic accidents, heart attacks, tuberculosis, hepatitis, acquired immune deficiency syndrome (AIDS), etc. These disorders are managed by the teaching or community hospitals.
- Repression of natural instincts—functional disorders, bulimia, anorexia, disorders of sexuality, depression, etc. These disorders are treatable by alternative modalities.

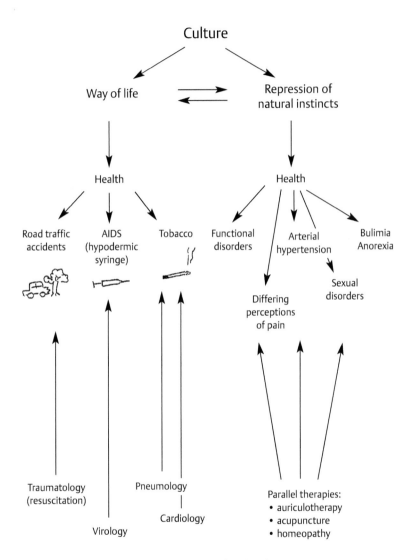

Fig. 2 The effects of cultural conditioning on health and medicine.

The Two Types of Ear Points

The concept of auriculotherapy is based on an understanding of the nature of the points.

It seems that on the ear there are two kinds of points:

1. Points linked directly to the nervous system (the pressure points)
These points are located with a pressure probe, and are painful when an organ is diseased.

In therapy, the points are treated with needles or massage (see **Figs. 3a, b**).

2. Neurohumoral-type points
These points are located by electrodetection and they are formed by specific structures—the neurovascular complexes.[1-3]

These points are treated with infrared lasers (see **Fig. 3c**).

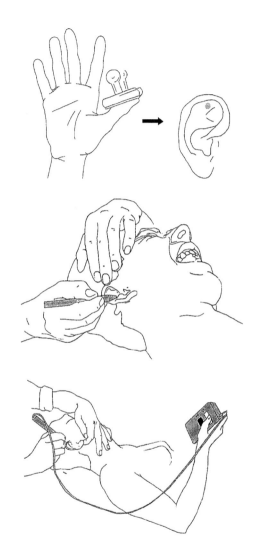

Fig. 3a–c

a A disorder in the body generates a pathological zone or point on the ear.

b Using the pain response to locate a pathological point on the ear (pressure probe).

c Using the Diascope to locate a pathological point on the ear (locating the neurovascular complexes). [4]

■ Points Linked Directly to the Nervous System: Reflex Points

These points are painful on pressure when a corresponding organ or region of the body is painful. This phenomenon is explained by the way in which the nervous system is organized.

The points on the ear are linked to various regions of the body through the spinothalamic and reticular systems. If a peripheral zone is distressed, the corresponding point on the ear point becomes sensitive, i.e., painful under pressure.

These reflex points are used to provide pain relief.

Fig. 4a, b   ▶

a Neurological basis of auricular reflex points.
b Locating sensitive ear points: The "grimace" sign.[4]

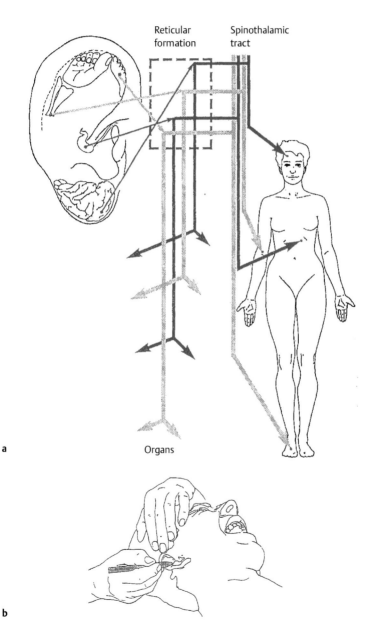

Reticular formation

Spinothalamic tract

a

Organs

b

▬ *Neurohumoral-Type Points: the Neurovascular Complexes*

J. E. H. Niboyet (1963) determined that:
- On the surface of the skin there are points of lower cutaneous electrical resistance (CER).
- These points are independent of skin secretions since they can be observed even after the skin has been thoroughly cleaned with a solution of alcohol, ether, and acetone.
- They correspond to acupuncture points described in Chinese medicine and can be detected on the body in living persons as well as cadavers.

From the work of Sénélar, Auziech, and Terral (1970–1980)
These authors studied the ear points with lower CER in humans and rabbits, and examined them under optical microscopy.

They have found specific histologic features under the points of lower CER, combining:
- An arteriole
- A venule
- A lymphatic vessel
- A free nerve ending

Myelin-sheathed nerve fibers are distributed among the vascular elements and may come into close proximity to the vascular structures.

This coexistence of nerves and thin-walled vessels in close proximity is not a random structuring, and we should note the release of hormonal or related factors by endocrine constituents following stimulation of the points. These formations are called **neurovascular complexes**.

- The neurohormonal points are detected by the use of instruments that measure variations in electrical resistance.
- They are detectable when there are peripheral functional disorders.
- These points can be treated by laser therapy.
- Some authors[5,6] have hypothesized that the neurovascular complexes have an active role in organ thermoregulation.

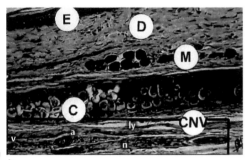

a

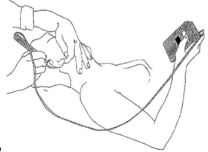

b

Fig. 5a, b Example of an ear "point" (magnified approximately × 300). [Reference 6, with permission of the author].

a E = Epidermis
   D = Dermis
   M = China ink
   C = Auricular cartilage
   CNV = Neurovascular complexes are consistently found in the tissue substrate below the points used in auriculotherapy (v, venule; a, arteriole; ly, lymphatic vessel; n, cutaneous nerve). The neurovascular structures have a relatively constant pattern.
b Using the Diascope to locate a pathological point on the ear (locating the neurovascular complexes). [4]

Anatomy of the Ear

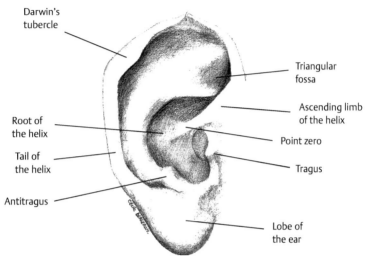

Darwin's tubercle

Triangular fossa

Ascending limb of the helix

Root of the helix

Point zero

Tail of the helix

Tragus

Antitragus

Lobe of the ear

a

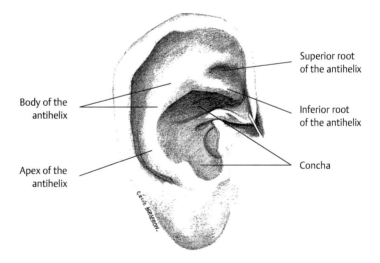

Superior root of the antihelix

Body of the antihelix

Inferior root of the antihelix

Apex of the antihelix

Concha

b

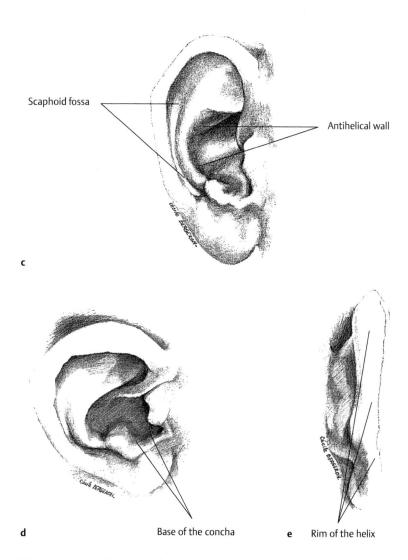

Scaphoid fossa

Antihelical wall

c

d

Base of the concha

e Rim of the helix

Fig. 6a–e Anatomy of the external ear.

Innervation of the Ear

There are four distinct zones on the external ear:
- **The central concha**—innervated by the parasympathetic fibers of the vagus nerve.
- **The middle auricle**—innervated by the mandibular branch of the trigeminal nerve (sympathetic fibers).
- **The helical-lobular region**—innervated by the superficial cervical plexus (mixed innervation).
- **The tragal region**—mixed innervation.

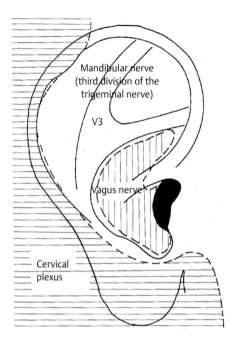

Fig. 7 Innervation of the ear according to J. Bossy,[7] by permission of the author.

Representation of the Organs on the Ear

The somatotopy of the ear is logical:
- **In the center**, the concha, innervated by the vagus nerve, contains the point locations of the tissues derived from the endoderm.
- **In the middle region**, the antihelix and a part of the helix innervated by the trigeminal nerve, contain the point locations of the tissues derived from the mesoderm.
- **In the peripheral area**, a part of the helix and the lobe innervated by the superficial cervical plexus contain the point locations of the tissues derived from the ectoderm.

Fig. 8a, b ▶
a Auricular locations (Paul Nogier, 1977).
b The auricle and the corresponding fetal image (Paul Nogier, 1969).

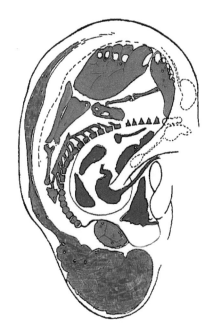

a

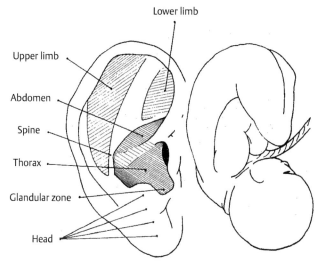

Lower limb

Upper limb

Abdomen

Spine

Thorax

Glandular zone

Head

b

Representation of the Vertebral Column

- The **spine** is represented on the antihelix.
- The **vertebral bodies** are represented on the antihelix ridge.
- The **muscles and ligaments** of the spine are represented on the exterior aspect of the antihelix.
- The **sympathetic chain** is represented on the antihelix wall.

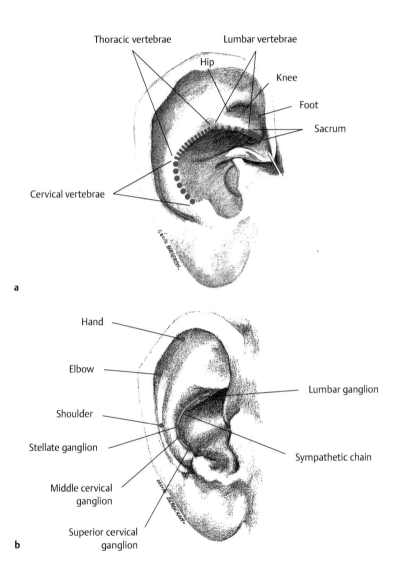

Fig. 9a, b Point locations of the limbs and the spinal column on the ear.

Ear Locations

- Mesodermic
- Endodermic
- Ectodermic

▬ Mesodermic Tissues

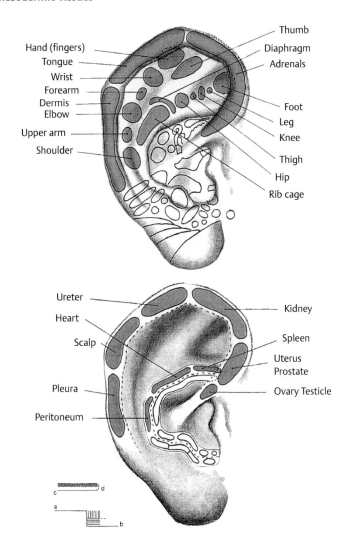

Fig. 10a, b Locations (Paul Nogier, 1987).
a Mesoderm: visible locations.
b Mesoderm: hidden locations.

■ Endodermic Tissues

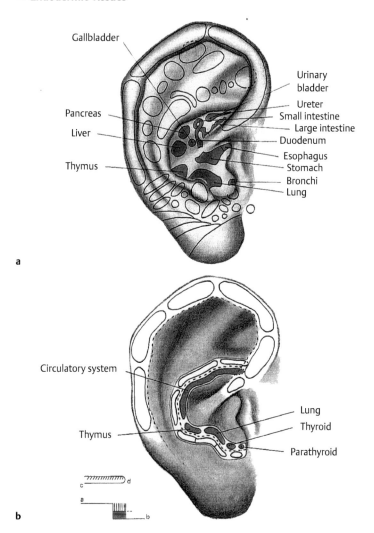

Fig. 11a, b Locations (Paul Nogier, 1987).
a Endoderm: visible locations.
b Endoderm: hidden locations.

Ectodermic Tissues

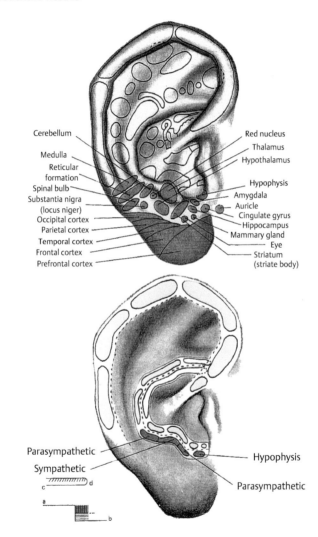

Cerebellum
Medulla
Reticular formation
Spinal bulb
Substantia nigra (locus niger)
Occipital cortex
Parietal cortex
Temporal cortex
Frontal cortex
Prefrontal cortex

Red nucleus
Thalamus
Hypothalamus
Hypophysis
Amygdala
Auricle
Cingulate gyrus
Hippocampus
Mammary gland
Eye
Striatum (striate body)

a

Parasympathetic
Sympathetic

Hypophysis

Parasympathetic

b

Fig. 12a, b Locations (Paul Nogier, 1987).
a Ectoderm: visible locations.
b Ectoderm: hidden locations.

Other Locations

Some points on the ear have a general effect. These points are known as **master points**.

- They are detectable mainly by means of electrodetection.
- They are best treated by infrared laser stimulation.
- Some organs are represented at more than one location on the ear. This is accounted for by the phase theory introduced by Paul Nogier in 1981. (See "Paul Nogier's Phase Theory," p. 106.)

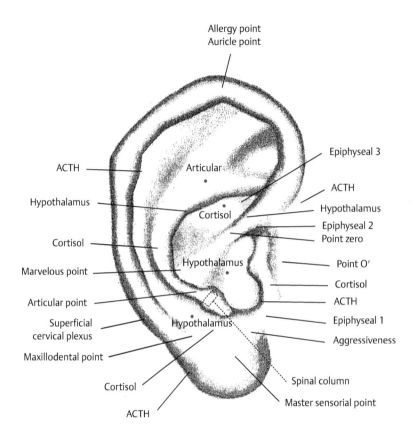

Fig. 13 Locations of some master points (Paul Nogier, 1987).

Methods of Point Detection

■ *Pressure (Pain) Detection*

Technique:
- **Palpation by hand**. The patient is lying on a table. The physician sits behind the patient and palpates both ears, searching for painful areas.
- **Eliciting the "grimace" sign** using a 250 g (blue) pressure probe.

Indications:
Indications for use of the pressure (pain) detection technique are peripheral disorders such as:
- Osteoarthritis
- Low back pain
- Gout (acute)
- Neuralgias

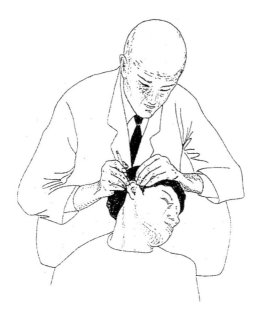

Fig. 14 Searching for points using a pressure probe.[4]

■ *Electrodetection*

Technique:
The procedure consists of locating a neurovascular complex in a pathological state. The instruments (punctoscope or electrodetector and stimulator [Agiscop DT]) utilize a differential measurement technique.

The instrument measures:
•   Skin resistance in the area surrounding point R1
•   Resistance of point R2
•   Resistance of the hand (RH)

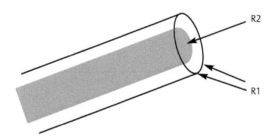

Fig. 15 Diagrammatic representation of an electrodetector.

When the relationship (RH–R1)/(RH–R2) varies from a value of 1, it indicates a drop in resistance at the point.

Caution: The accuracy of electrodetection is affected by:
- Ingestion of certain medications (such as cortisone or high doses of nonsteroi-dal anti-inflammatory drugs [NSAIDs])
- Low atmospheric pressure

Indications:
Indications for electrodetection include:
- Chronic pain
- Functional disorders
- Psychological problems
- Tobacco addiction

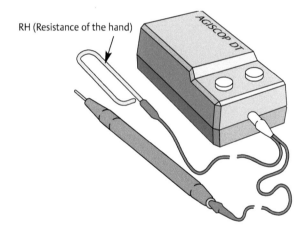

RH (Resistance of the hand)

Fig. 16 Agiscop DT

Point Treatment Methods

Treatment of points detected with a pressure probe:
- Massage the points with a glass rod.
- Standard (non-intradermal) needles—retain for 20 minutes.
- Semipermanent needles—small needles are retained in the ear for several days.*
- Laser—each point should be treated at the frequency related to its specific location, i.e., zone A, B, C, D, E, F, or G (see **Figs. 18a, b**).

Treatment of points located by electrodetection:
- Mostly by laser
- Also by needles, semipermanent needles, or electric current.

---

* The ASP (aiguille semi permanente) system (using permanent needles) was introduced by Paul Nogier in 1973.

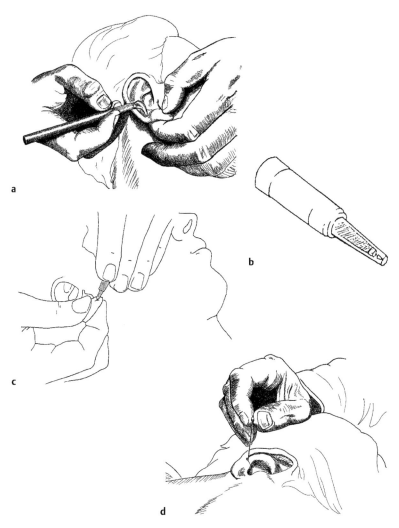

Fig. 17a–d

a Auricular massage technique.
b Semipermanent needle (SEDATELEC Irigny France, see p. 165).[4]
c Inserting a semipermanent needle.[4]
d Auricular needling technique.

Indications for Auriculotherapy

Pain:
- Metabolic
- Traumatic
- Neurological

Functional disorders:
- Tachycardia
- Constipation
- Irritable bowel syndrome
- Chronic fatigue
- Menstrual problems such as amenorrhea or dysmenorrhea

Disorders of dependency:
- Tobacco addiction
- Benzodiazepine (tranquilizer) use
- Antidepressant use

Psychological disorders:
- Reactive depression
- Anxiety

Dermatologic disorders:
- Eczema
- Psoriasis
- Alopecia

Contraindications:
- Pregnancy

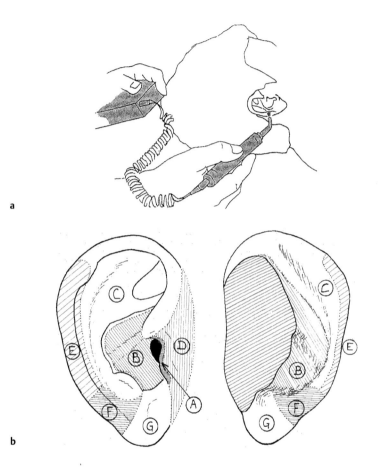

Fig. 18a, b
a Ear point treatment with a pulsed infrared laser device.
b The different zones for auricular laser treatment. The points are treated at the zone-specific frequency.[4]

■ *Tobacco Addiction Treatment Protocol*

In my opinion, every smoker is a depressive person who is unaware of their depression. **Nicotine is an antidepressant**.

Treatment:
- Evaluate the level of dependence on tobacco.
- Only treat smokers who are motivated and emotionally stable. Decline to treat any individual who is clearly unbalanced or psychotic.
- See the patient in the morning before they have smoked the first cigarette of the day.
- Treat the right ear in right-handed and the left ear in left-handed individuals.
- Locate the points with an electrodetector.
- Instruct the patient to stimulate the needles and to eat a healthy diet.
- See the patient on a regular basis to prevent possible weight gain, relapse or psychological problems.

Result:
- It is not that hard to stop smoking, the real challenge is not starting smoking again.
- We have observed the following rate of success after:
    - 1 month: 85%
    - 1 year: 36%
    - 2 years: 15%

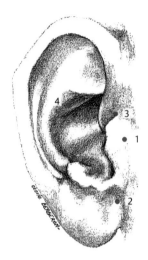

Fig. 19 Tobacco addiction treatment protocol: points to treat.
1 Point 0'
2 Aggressiveness
3 Pharynx (throat)
4 Point for the stimulation of the sympathetic system: point situated on the antihelical wall.

■ *Treatment of Toxic Scars*

A scar is toxic when it causes apparently unrelated problems such as:
- Chronic fatigue
- Eczema
- Hypotension
- Allergies
- Migraines
- Headaches

Toxic scars are often:
- Horizontal
- Red
- Paresthetic

Treatment:
- Auriculotherapy treatment is very effective.
- The points should be treated with standard (non-intradermal) needles, retained for 20 minutes. The patient should be seen on a weekly basis for about 6 months.

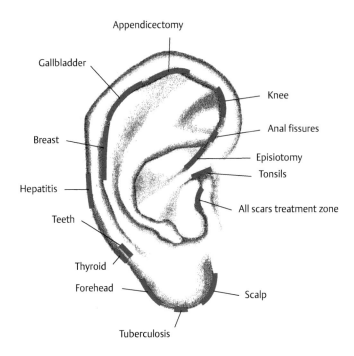

Fig. 20 Points for the treatment of toxic scars.

■ *Obesity*

Auriculotherapy is not appropriate as a treatment for endocrine disorders. On the other hand, a number of laboratory and clinical studies have proved that needles in the ear stimulate the hypothalamic nucleus and enhance the sensation of satiety.

Auriculotherapy can thus be utilized in the struggle against obesity.

Treatment:
Points to needle:
▶ Anterior and posterior stomach points
▶ Hypothalamus points
▶ Hunger (commissure) point

The auriculotherapy treatment is delivered combined with a simple diet plan. The patient should be seen every 15 days.

1. Semi-free choice diet

Breakfast
• Tea or coffee with a little "half and half" cream, but no sugar
• Two or three slices of a six-grain bread with a little butter

10 – 10:30 am
• One or two apples, or
• One small cup of strawberries or raspberries

Lunch
- A salad, selected from:
  - Radishes
  - Lettuce
  - Tomatoes
  - Cucumber
  - Endives
  - Beans
- With a dressing of:
  - Nonfat yoghurt, creamed
  - Mustard
  - Lemon
  - Garlic
  - Kitchen herbs
  - One teaspoon of olive or sunflower oil
- One fillet of fish, steamed or boiled
- One hot steamed vegetable, served with- out butter, such as:
  - Artichokes
  - Beans
  - Italian squash
  - Spinach
  - Ratatouille (a traditional French vegetable stew consisting of onions, egg- plant, zucchini, tomatoes, and peppers)
  - Asparagus
- **No peas or carrots**
- **No bread, starchy foods, fruit, or wine**

4 – 4:30 pm
- An apple or a pear

Dinner
- One or two slices of ham with the fat removed
  or
- One egg cooked without butter
- A salad with a yoghurt dressing
- A hot vegetable
- **No garden peas or carrots**
- **No bread, starchy foods, fruit, or wine**

2. 1500 calories per day diet

Breakfast
- Whole milk with tea or coffee (250 mL)
- Butter (5 g)
- Bread (40 g)

Lunch
- Vegetable bouillon
- Grilled steak (150 g)
- Green beans (200 g)
- Potatoes (100 g)
- Butter or oil
- Apples (200 g)

Dinner
- Cooked endives (200 g)
- Eggs (1)
- Gruyere cheese (50 g)
- Pear (1)

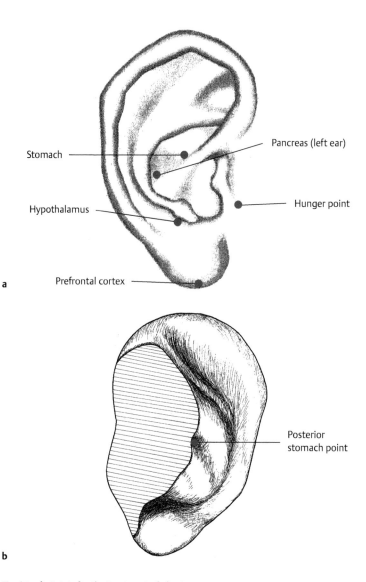

Stomach

Pancreas (left ear)

Hypothalamus

Hunger point

Prefrontal cortex

a

Posterior
stomach point

b

Fig. 21a, b Points for the treatment of obesity.

▬ *Constipation*

Fewer than two bowel movements per week indicate constipation.

Treatment:
- The patient should return for auriculotherapy every 15 days. The points should be treated with semipermanent needles.
- Points to needle:
  - Large intestine on the left and right ears
  - Gallbladder on the anterior and posterior aspects of the right ear
  - Hypothalamus points
- It is also essential that the patient consumes a diet rich in fiber and a therapeutic drink rich in magnesium, and undertakes regular, daily exercise such as walking.
- The patient should go to the bathroom at the same time every day, and avoid taking laxatives, since they simply maintain the tendency toward constipation.

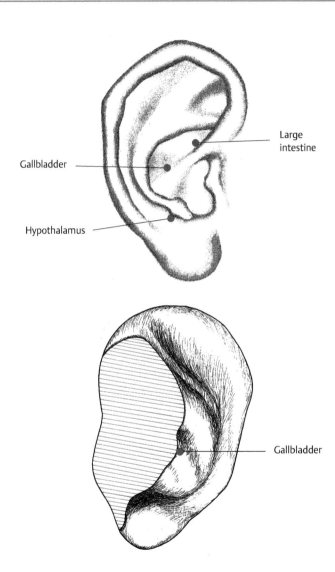

Fig. 22a, b Points for the treatment of constipation.

■ *Sciatica*

"Sciatica is not an inevitable disease."[8] It is frequently the result of articular constriction between the vertebrae, initiated by postural problems. However, we know that human posture is linked to tension in the paravertebral muscles—which are themselves dependent on information received from various receptors, principally in the:
- Eyes
- Jaw
- Feet
- Skin

A problem with any of these receptors (ocular movement disorder, malocclusion, flat feet, scars, etc.) can initiate spasms in the paravertebral muscles, which over the long term develop regional constrictions.

Treatment:
In a case of sciatica:
- Treat the pain with:
  - Point L5–S1
  - Point zero
  - Point O'
- Treat the cause with:
  - Eye point
  - Jaw point
  - Scar point
- Treat the consequences with:
  - The cervical points in particular (first cervical is often affected)

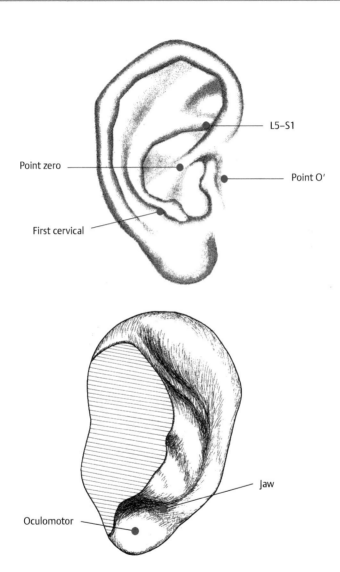

Fig. 23a, b Points for the treatment of sciatica.

▪ *Female Infertility*

Female infertility is a frequent reason for consultation with an auriculotherapist.

Some women with normal biologic and radiologic test results are unable to conceive.

Treatment:
In treating such cases, we must proceed through several stages.

1. Eliminate any nutritional allergies. A hidden allergy can indirectly cause lesions in the jejunum of the small intestine and thereby generate micro and trace element deficiencies, which are harmful for the nervous system.
2. Treat any evident toxic scars.
- Give auriculotherapy treatment 15 days before the next menstruation is due to start. The points to treat are likely to be from the following:
    - Prefrontal cortex
    - Hypothalamus
    - Hypophysis
    - Point O'
    - Ovaries
    - Liver
- Treatments should be given monthly.

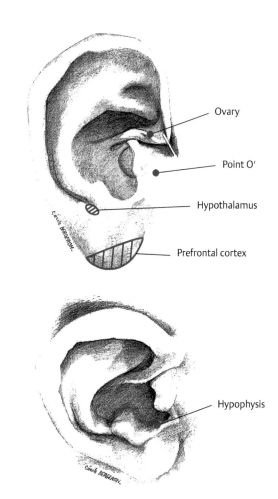

Ovary

Point O′

Hypothalamus

Prefrontal cortex

a

Hypophysis

b

Fig. 24a, b Points for the treatment of female infertility.

▬ *Spasmophilia (Latent Tetany)*

Spasmophilia (latent tetany) is a disease that primarily affects women. Frequent treatment is needed over a protracted period.

Treatment:
- The organism's ionic balance must be restored to equilibrium. To accomplish this the exchanges that take place at the level of the intestinal barrier need to be facilitated. We must therefore look for one or more nutritional allergies. The one most frequently found is an allergy to milk products. In most cases, patients are advised to avoid consumption of any dairy foods (milk, cheese, yoghurt, and other milk derivatives) for several months.
- Small doses of magnesium, manganese, copper, and lithium should be taken in trace element (oligoelement) form.
- Auriculotherapy treatment is two-pronged. Treat:
  - Point O', left and right
  - Adrenal points, left and right, using semipermanent needles

Caution: Do not confuse a malabsorption syndrome caused by nutritional allergies with an anxiety disorder.

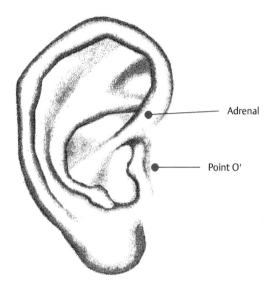

Fig. 25 Points for the treatment of spasmophilia (latent tetany).

■ *Shingles (Herpes Zoster)*

Pain due to shingles can be relieved very quickly with auriculotherapy. The points should be located with a pressure probe.

Treatment:
- The most impressive results are seen when the patient is treated within the first few hours of onset of the condition.
  - The affected dermatome is identified (i.e., D6).
  - Point zero is needled and the D6 radius vector is treated. This is an imaginary line originating at point zero and passing through the D6 point on the antihelix.
  - Painful points along the course of the line are identified with a pressure probe and standard needles inserted at these locations. Remember to explore the antihelix wall and the helix rim.
- Once the crisis has passed, try to determine why the patient contracted the disease.

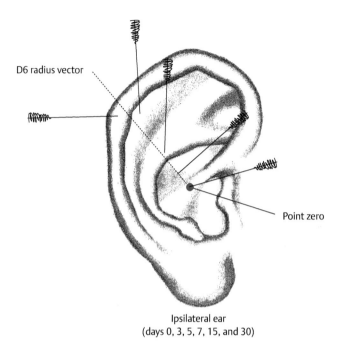

Ipsilateral ear
(days 0, 3, 5, 7, 15, and 30)

Fig. 26 Points for the treatment of shingles (herpes zoster).

■ *Reflex Sympathetic Dystrophy (Shoulder–Hand Syndrome)*

Reflexive algodystrophy manifests as pain and circulatory problems caused by re-flex arterial vasoconstriction following trauma.

Treatment:
This painful and chronic disease can be relieved by needling certain points in the ear.
- In algodystrophy of the upper limb:
  - Stellate ganglion point on the anterior antihelix wall on the C7 radius vec-tor, located using an electrosensor
  - Shoulder and hand points, located with a pressure probe
- In algodystrophy of the lower limb:
  - Lumbar sympathetic ganglion, located on the L1–L2 radius vector on the anterior antihelix wall, identified by electrodetection
  - Hip and foot points
- Treatment should be given every 15 days.
- Infrared laser pulsed over the locus dolendi at frequencies A, B, E, G is benefi-cial as complementary treatment.

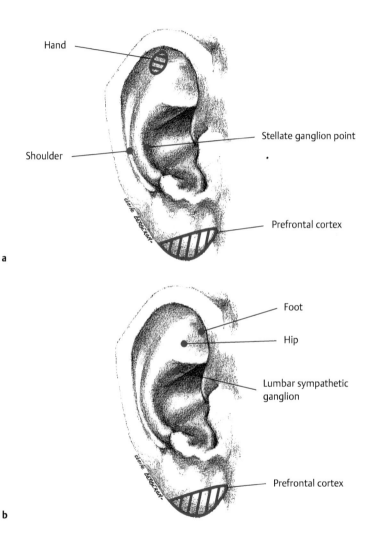

Fig. 27a, b Points for the treatment of reflex sympathetic dystrophy.
a Algodystrophy of the upper limb.
b Algodystrophy of the lower limb.

■ *Shoulder Pain*

Shoulder disorders are common and respond very well to auriculotherapy.

Treatment:
- Identify and treat any **dental focus**. Check for:
    - Apical granulomas
    - Cysts
    - Electro galvanism between two different metals in the mouth
    - Impacted wisdom teeth
- Examine the **ipsilateral ear** in the region of:
    - The maxillary point
    - The shoulder point
    - The eye point
    - Trigeminal nerve point
    - Point O′
    - Point zero
    - Stellate ganglion point
- **If an infrared laser is available**, the painful area of the shoulder can be irradiated at frequencies A and E.

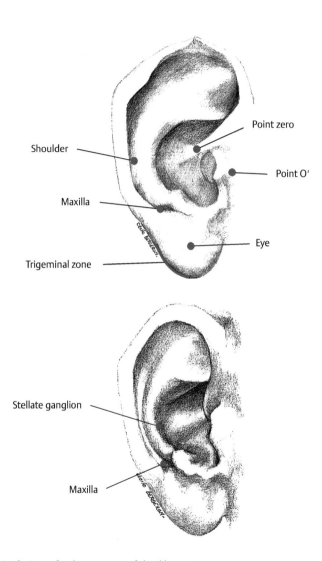

Fig. 28a, b Points for the treatment of shoulder pain.

■ *Geriatric Spinal Disorders*

Auriculotherapy is a superior technique for osteoarthritic disorders in older people. Used by itself, it can prevent the need for anti-inflammatory and analgesic drugs.

Treatment:
Treatments should be regular—generally monthly, and in some cases every 2 weeks.
- Point O′: left and right. These two points are located with the Agiscop.
- The antitragus and antihelix points can be examined bilaterally with a pressure probe. Use standard (non-intradermal) needles and retain for about 20 minutes.

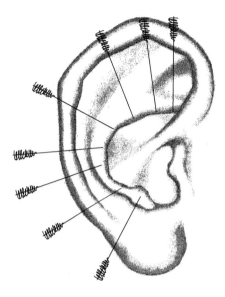

Fig. 29 Points for the treatment of geriatric spinal disorders.

▪ Fibrocystic Breast Disease and Mastodynia (Painful Breasts)

Mastopathies are very common in Western countries. In France, 1 in 10 women will develop breast cancer, whereas in China this figure is 1 in 80. Many women suffer with fibrocystic breast disease and mastodynia.

Treatment:
The points to treat are:
- **Liver**: on the right ear, located by electrodetection
- **Hypothalamus**: right or left ear, located with electrodetection
- **Hypophysis**: concha base, right or left ear, located by electrodetection
- **Breast**: on the lobe, located by pressure probe
- **Ovary**: located by electrodetection

The treatment should be given every month.

Remember to prescribe a dietary regimen:
Foods to be avoided: milk, cheese, yoghurt, and other dairy-related foods; beef and veal; and coffee and tea.

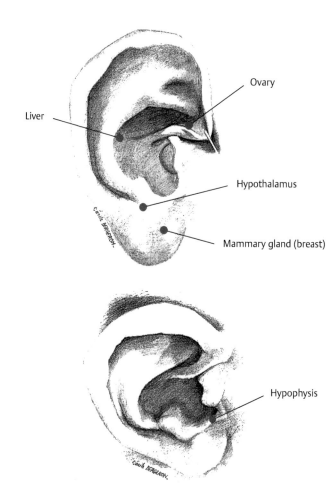

Fig. 30a, b Points for the treatment of fibrocystic breast disease and mastodynia (painful breasts).

■ *Migraines*

Although hard to treat successfully with conventional medical treatments, migraines are often relieved or cured with auriculotherapy.

Treatment:
- **Identify any oculomotor dysfunction** and treat it either by auriculotherapy or by re-education with eye exercises.
- **Treat toxic scars as needed** (see p. 34)
- **Treat any dental foci:** The term dental focus refers to a painful or painless dental pathology which gives rise to apparently unrelated symptoms.
- **Treat first rib syndrome if indicated.**
- **Eliminate any nutritional allergy** or pseudoallergy.
- **Check the following points:**
  - On the **posterior aspect** of the auricle:
    Eye point
    Jaw point
    First cervical vertebra
    First rib point
    Pelvis point
  - On the **anterior aspect** of the auricle:
    Point O'
    Eye point
    Maxilla
    Thalamus
    Hypothalamus
    Liver, on the right ear
    Pancreas on the left ear

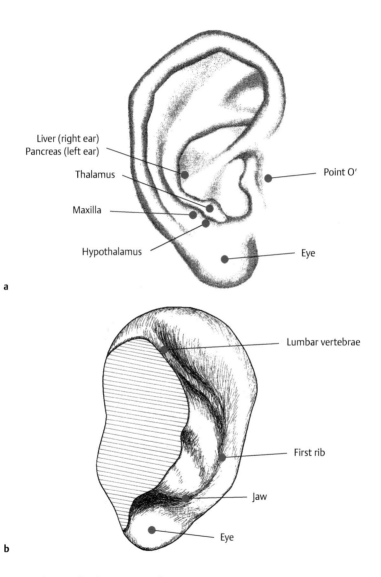

Liver (right ear)
Pancreas (left ear)

Thalamus

Maxilla

Hypothalamus

Point O′

Eye

a

Lumbar vertebrae

First rib

Jaw

Eye

b

Fig. 31a, b Points for the treatment of migraines.

▬ *Depressive Disorders*

Three types of depression are amenable to treatment by auricular reflexotherapy.

1. Reactive depression
Treatment:
Reactive depression needs early treatment. The points needled are:
- E points: They are needled in rapid succession, the needles are retained for 1 second
- Point O': right and left ear with semipermanent needles
- Prefrontal cortex point: with semipermanent needles (see **Fig. 32b**)

2. Seasonal affect depression (SAD)
SAD is primarily encountered during the winter, manifesting as sadness and weight gain.

Treatment:
The hypophysis point on the right or left ear using a semipermanent needle.

The patient is prescribed 30 minutes of exposure to strong bright light daily, at a regular fixed time (see **Fig. 32a**).

3. Postpartum depression
Popularly known as the "baby blues," postpartum depression is frequently the result of a toxic scar on the perineum. Treatment is by two needles tangential on the ascending limb of the helix (see **Fig. 32c**).

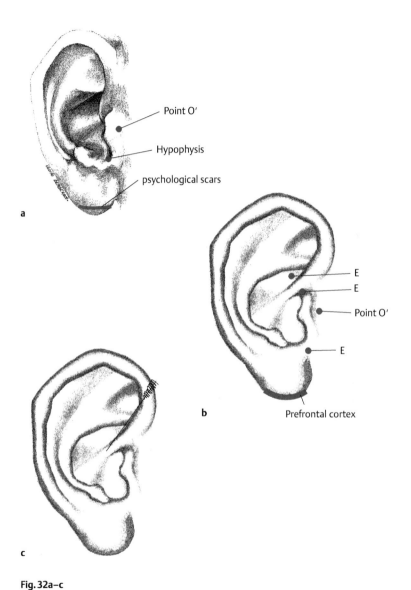

Fig. 32a–c
a Points for the treatment of seasonal affect disorder (SAD).
b, c Points for the treatment of reactive depression.

▰ *First Rib Syndrome*

Keep in mind:
Strictly speaking, the syndrome is not an indication for auriculotherapy—it is considered actually an obstacle to auricular treatment. The head of the first rib is displaced following some trauma or physical strain and mechanically irritates the stellate ganglion, giving rise to a wide range of pathologies:
*   Frequent urgent diarrhea (due to accelerated intestinal transit)
*   Headaches
*   Visual problems
*   Blood pressure problems
*   Thoracic oppression
*   Trigeminal neuralgia
*   Reflexive algodystrophy of the upper limbs

Diagnosis:
A diagnosis of first rib syndrome is based on three criteria:
*   Existence of a probable cervical trauma
*   Pain on palpation of the first rib
*   Asymmetry in the right and left radial pulses. This is due to arterial stress induced by adrenergic impulses

Treatment:
The first rib should be repositioned either manually or by prescribed exercises.

Location of the auriculotherapy points:
*   On the posterior aspect of the auricle—the first rib point
*   On the anterior aspect of the antihelix wall, right side radius vector C7—the stellate ganglion point

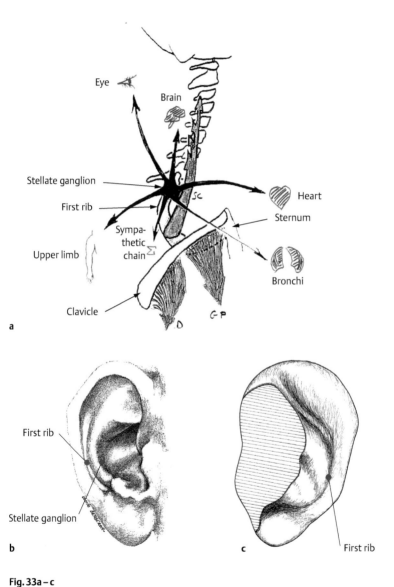

Fig. 33a – c
a The first rib.
b, c Points for the treatment of first rib syndrome.

■ *Hypotension*

Hypotension is a symptom often found among women who also display symptoms similar to nutrition-related pathology, such as headaches, constipation, fatigue, spasmophilia, etc.

Examination of a hypotensive patient:
- Evaluate the skin texture—is it fine or thick?
- Is there any mottled discoloration on the thighs?

These two signs are suggestive of an allergy to dairy proteins.

Treatment:
Treat any evident toxic scars (see p. 34).
- Auricular locations:
    - Thumb point—this has a hypertensive action
    - Sympathetic point on the anterior antihelix wall
    - Liver point
    - Hypothalamus point
- Dietary recommendations:
    - Eat licorice candy periodically.
    - Drink mineral water with added salt.

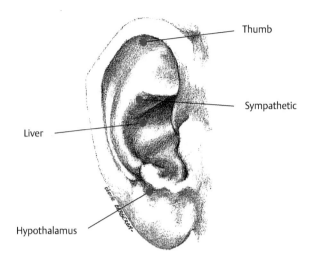

Thumb

Sympathetic

Liver

Hypothalamus

Fig. 34 Points for the treatment of hypotension.

■ *Food Allergies*

Dietary allergies affect large numbers of people. Since the majority of dietary allergies are hidden, with barely noticeable or no symptoms, it is not uncommon for a person to be unaware of them.

General symptoms
- Fatigue, with occasional sudden episodes of somnolence
- Appetite dysfunction

Gastrointestinal
- Reduced motility
- Intestinal pain
- Foul-smelling flatulence
- Diarrhea or constipation
- Anal pruritus

Articular
- Idiomatic joint pains

Gynecologic
- Painful breasts
- Premenstrual syndrome
- Libidinal dysfunction

Neurological
- Migraines
- General headaches
- Anxiety attacks
- Spasmophilia/tetany
- Depression

Dermatologic
- Tendency to acne
- Hair loss—partial or total
- Eczema
- Urticaria triggered by exposure to sunshine

Cardiovascular
- Tachycardia
- Blood pressure—elevated or depressed
- Edema in the lower limbs
- Pulmonary
- Asthma
- Bronchitis

Diagnosis is by avoidance followed by reintroduction of suspected food items.

Treatment:
Treatment is to stop consuming the allergen. The prime offenders are: food colorings, food preservatives, grains, milk products, citrus fruits, tomatoes, tea, coffee, and eggs.

Treat the following auricular points:
- Liver point
- Pancreas point
- Large intestine point
- Point O'
- Hypothalamus point
- Allergy point

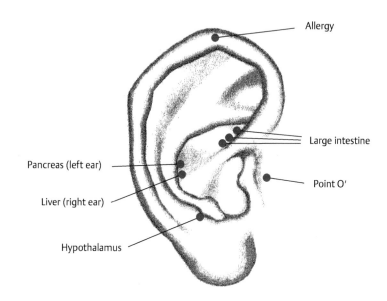

Fig. 35 Points for the treatment of dietary allergies.

■ *Cerebral Laterality Disorders*

Each auricle corresponds to the opposite cerebral hemisphere.

Basic concepts:
- In a right-handed person, the left hemisphere of the brain controls logical, abstract, and mathematical thinking.
- The right hemisphere controls vision, hearing, and artistic and empirical thinking.
- 90% of people are true right-handers—their language center is in the left hemisphere.
- 1% are true left-handers—their language center is in the right hemisphere.
- 9% are poorly lateralized left-handers—their language center is in the left hemisphere.
- Animals do not display hemispherical lateralization.
- Asymmetry is an anatomic concept.
- Laterality is a functional concept.

Pathology:
- Hyperactivity of the right hemisphere:
  - Hypersensitivity, hyperactivity, anxiety, anguish, and depression may be seen following psychologic trauma, trauma to the frontal area of the brain, or after giving up cigarette smoking.
- Hyperactivity of the left hemisphere:
  - Abstract thinking divorced from practical reality, the manic phase in bipolar disorder, psychotic states.

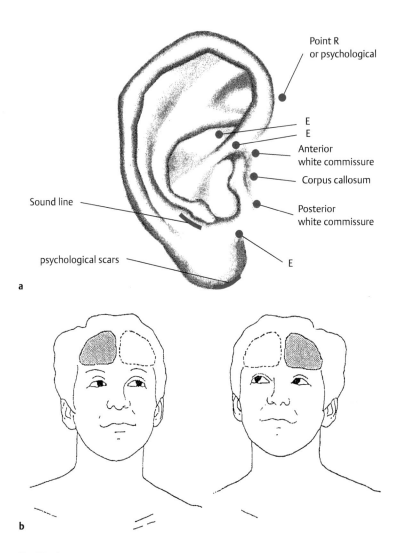

Fig. 36a, b
a Points or zones to explore in patients with cerebral laterality disorders.
b The direction of the gaze is deviated to the side opposite the functioning hemisphere.[4]

■ *Psoriasis*

Viewed as neurodermatitis by some and dermoneurosis by others, psoriasis remains an enigma in terms of its physiopathology.

Treatment:
Treatment by auriculo-acupuncture can sometimes produce remarkable results. The patient should be treated weekly for a total of 30–40 sessions. It usually takes at least 15 treatments before improvement is seen.

Points to check and treat:
- Point O′
- Liver point
- Psychic scars
- Helix rim points

The helix rim points should be needled slightly in posterior position as shown in **Fig. 37a**.

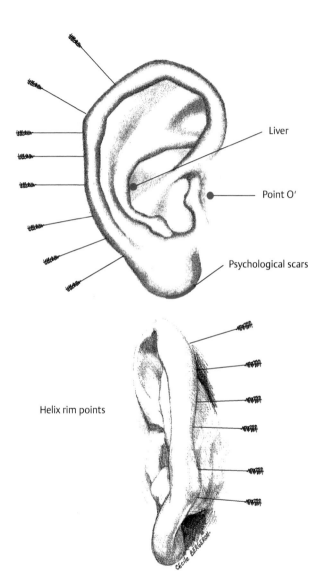

a

Liver

Point O′

Psychological scars

Helix rim points

b

Cécile BERGERON.

Fig. 37a, b Points for the treatment of psoriasis.

■ *Trigeminal Neuralgia*

This sometimes excruciatingly painful disorder is often amenable to treatment by auriculotherapy.

Treatment:
- Treat as for first rib syndrome if necessary (see p. 62):
    - With manipulation
    - And auriculotherapy points
      first rib
      stellate ganglion
- Treat any existing dental problems:
    - With dental treatment
    - By needling:
      dental points on the ear
- Needle tangentially to the border of the lobe on the side opposite to the pain.
- Thalamus point (antitragus) ipsilaterally.
- If possible treat with infrared laser at A, B, E, and C frequencies over the painful trigeminal zone.

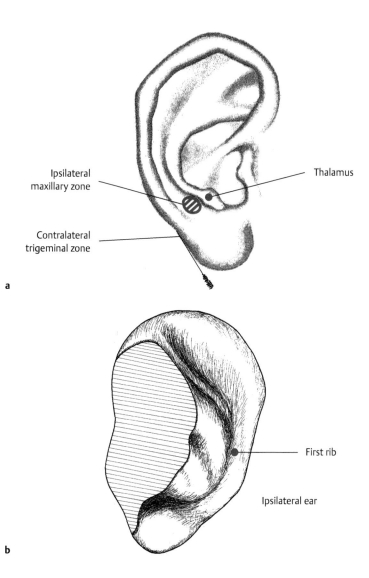

Fig. 38a, b Points for the treatment of trigeminal neuralgia.

▬ *Acute Hemorrhoids*

Auriculotherapy treatment of acute hemorrhoids is frequently extremely success-ful, since the pain and bleeding may recede rapidly.

Treatment:
The following dietary and sanitary rules should be observed:
- Avoid hot baths and showers.
- Take regular, daily walks.
- Wash with cold water after every bowel movement.
- Avoid:
    - Pork
    - Coffee
    - Tea
    - Pepper and spices
    - Alcohol

Auriculotherapy points:
- Hemorrhoid points located in the cymba concha
- Sacral sympathetic point
- Hypothalamus point

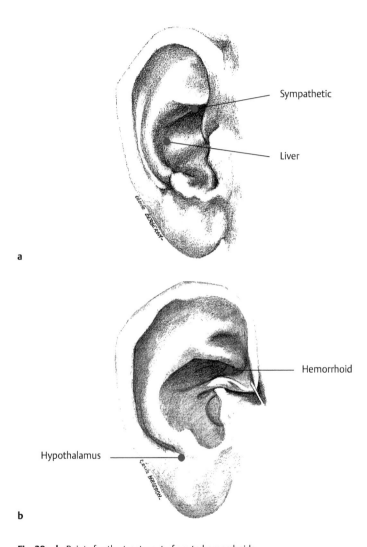

Fig. 39a, b Points for the treatment of acute hemorrhoids.

▬ Anguish and Anxiety

Anxiety is unfocused fear, anguish is anxiety somatized.

Some ideas to keep in mind:
- Certain animals are anxious by nature.
- Anguish stems from autonomic nervous system involvement.
- Anxiety and anguish are not inevitably symptomatic of a psychic disorder.

Some recommendations:
- The diet should be adapted to the individual with anxiety. Certain foods can trigger allergies, e.g., dairy products, grains, eggs, tomatoes, and chocolate. Other foods contain active principles that can escalate feelings of anxiety, e.g.:
  - Certain alcoholic beverages
  - Crustaceans
  - Food preservatives
  - Artificial food coloring
- Avoid prescribing antidepressants if at all possible; the symptoms simply become masked without resolution of the problem.
- Check for a physical source of the anxiety, e.g.:
  - Thoracic outlet syndrome
  - Spinal problems
  - Hiatal hernia
  - Coccygeal misalignment

Treatment:
Treat with auriculotherapy on a regular basis using the following points:
- Eye point
- Subcortical points
- Antihelix points
- Stomach
- Allergy point
- Cortex points
- Antihelix anterior wall points
- Point O'
- Kidney
- Pancreas

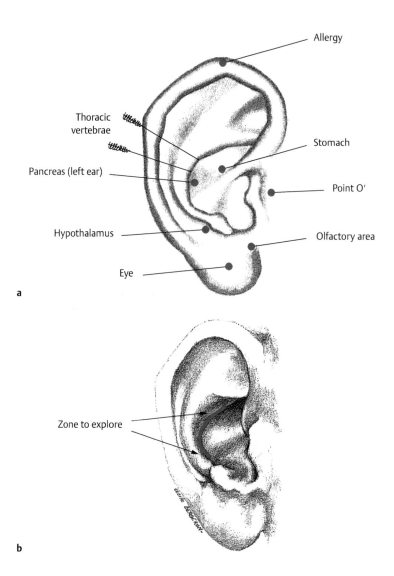

Fig. 40a, b Points for the treatment of anguish and anxiety.

■ *Pediatric Hyperactivity*

Look for a dietary source of the condition. The most common causes are listed below:

- Food colorings and preservatives (79%)
- Soy (73%)
- Cow's milk (64%)
- Chocolate (59%)
- Grapes/raisins (50%)
- Wheat (49%)
- Oranges (45%)
- Cheese from cow's milk (40%)
- Chicken eggs (39%)
- Peanuts (32%)
- Corn (29%)
- Fish (23%)
- Oats (23%)
- Melon (21%)
- Tomatoes (20%)
- Ham (20%)

(Adapted from Joseph Egger.[9])

Treatment:
The auriculotherapy points to use are:

- Allergy point
- Liver point
- Pancreas point
- Aggressiveness point
- Point O'
- Point R
- Prefrontal cortex point

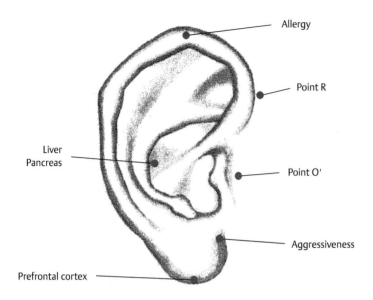

Fig. 41 Points for the treatment of pediatric hyperactivity.

■ *Chronic Progressive Polyarthritis*

The treatment approach is two-pronged.

1. Dietary
The following foods are most likely to aggravate polyarthritis.[10]
(Numbers in brackets refer to the percentage of sensitive individuals.)

Foods (Sensitive individuals %)
- Corn (56%)
- Wheat (54%)
- Pork (39%)
- Oranges (39%)
- Milk (37%)
- Oats (37%)
- Rye (34%)
- Eggs (32%)
- Beef (32%)
- Coffee (27%)
- Barley (24%)
- Cheese (24%)
- Grapefruit (24%)
- Tomatoes (20%)
- Nuts (20%)
- Cane sugar (17%)
- Butter (17%)
- Lamb (17%)

2. Anti-inflammatory points to treat every 15 days
- ACTH point
- Cortisol point
- Allergy point
- Liver point
- Pancreas point

Treatment:
- The ACTH and cortisol points are treated for only a second with standard (non-intradermal) needles.
- Treatment of polyarthritis with needles does not preclude concurrent ortho-dox treatment with anti-inflammatory drugs and gold salts.

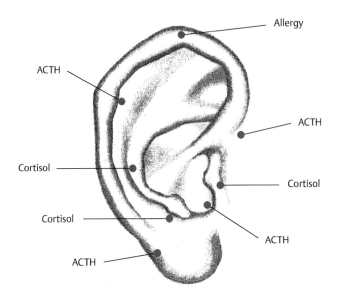

Fig. 42 Points for the treatment of chronic progressive polyarthritis.

▬ *Asthma*

Whatever the root cause might be, it is important to keep in mind that dietary choices may be determining factors in the cure of asthma.

The most frequently implicated foods according to D. G. Wraith[11]

Below 15 years of age:
- Milk (58%)
- Eggs (36%)
- Food coloring (33%)
- Wheat (6%)
- Others (35%)
  (cheese, fish, chocolate, soy, citrus fruits, chicken, hazelnuts, maize, oats, rye)

Above 15 years of age:
- Milk (59%)
- Eggs (20%)
- Wheat (32%)
- Food coloring (11%)
- Preservatives (10%)
- Others (63%)

The principle points indicated:
- Liver point
- Pancreas point
- Point O′
- Bronchial point
- Allergy point

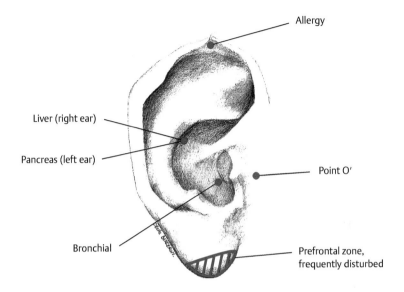

Fig. 43 Points for the treatment of asthma.

Anatomy of the Posterior Ear

The posterior surface of the auricle is also known as the mastoidal surface. It has a smaller surface area than the anterior aspect and has two significant grooves.

The cephalo-auricular groove:
This groove defines the border between the cranium and the auricle. The temple tips of spectacles rest in this groove. An important depression lies at the center of this groove—the central posterior fossa.

The posterior antihelix groove:
This groove runs vertically over the back of the auricle.

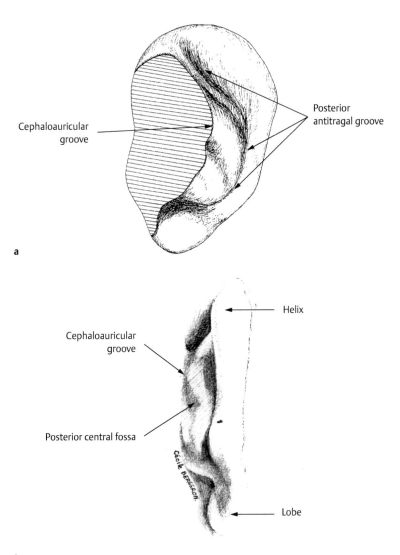

Fig. 44 Anatomy of the posterior ear.

Mesodermic Locations on the Posterior Surface of the Ear

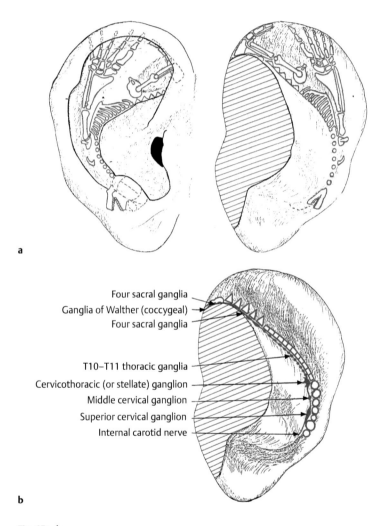

Fig. 45a, b
a Osteoarticular somatotopy according to René Bourdiol.
b Representation of the latero-vertebral ganglia on the mastoidal surface of the ear according to René Bourdiol.[7]

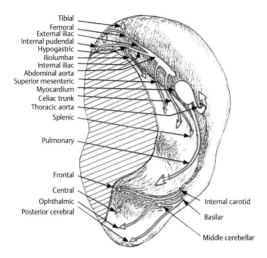

a

Tibial
Femoral
External iliac
Internal pudendal
Hypogastric
Iliolumbar
Internal iliac
Abdominal aorta
Superior mesenteric
Myocardium
Celiac trunk
Thoracic aorta
Splenic
Pulmonary
Frontal
Central
Ophthalmic
Posterior cerebral

Internal carotid
Basilar
Middle cerebellar

b

Inferior hyoid
Anterior vertebral
Lateral vertebral (anterior)
Lateral vertebral (posterior)
Superior hyoid
Neck, all
Cephalogyric*
Floor of the mouth
Tongue

Occipital
Frontal
Periorbital and palpebral
Muscles of the nose
Buccal and peribuccal muscles

* (muscles that flex, extend, and rotate the neck, and raise the shoulders)

Fig. 46a, b

a Cardio-arterial representation on the mastoidal surface of the ear according to René Bourdiol.[7]

b Representation of the muscles of the face and neck on the mastoidal surface of the ear according to René Bourdiol.[7]

Endodermic Locations on the Posterior Surface of the Ear

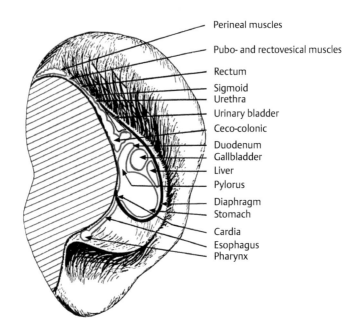

Perineal muscles

Pubo- and rectovesical muscles

Rectum

Sigmoid
Urethra
Urinary bladder
Ceco-colonic

Duodenum
Gallbladder
Liver
Pylorus

Diaphragm
Stomach

Cardia
Esophagus
Pharynx

a

▲

Fig. 47a–c ▶

a The digestive system represented on the right mastoidal surface according to René Bourdiol.[7]

b The digestive system represented on the left mastoidal surface according to René Bourdiol.[7]

c The respiratory system represented on the mastoidal surface according to René Bourdiol.[7]

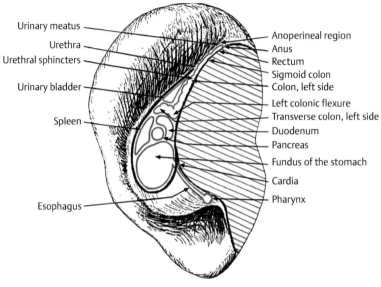

Urinary meatus
Urethra
Urethral sphincters
Urinary bladder
Spleen
Esophagus

Anoperineal region
Anus
Rectum
Sigmoid colon
Colon, left side
Left colonic flexure
Transverse colon, left side
Duodenum
Pancreas
Fundus of the stomach
Cardia
Pharynx

b

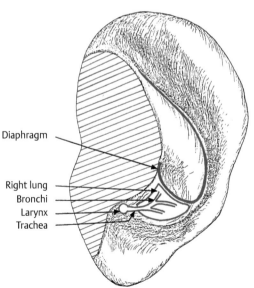

Diaphragm
Right lung
Bronchi
Larynx
Trachea

c

Ectodermic Locations on the Posterior Surface of the Ear

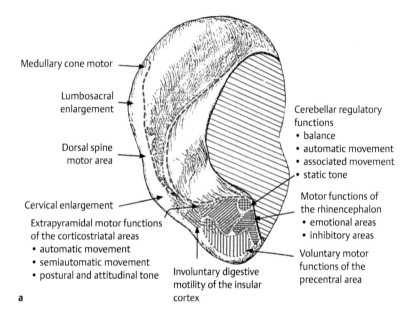

Medullary cone motor

Lumbosacral enlargement

Dorsal spine motor area

Cervical enlargement

Extrapyramidal motor functions of the corticostriatal areas
• automatic movement
• semiautomatic movement
• postural and attitudinal tone

Cerebellar regulatory functions
• balance
• automatic movement
• associated movement
• static tone

Motor functions of the rhinencephalon
• emotional areas
• inhibitory areas

Voluntary motor functions of the precentral area

Involuntary digestive motility of the insular cortex

a

▲
Fig. 48a–d

▶

a Auricular representation of motor functions according to René Bourdiol.[7]
b Auricular representation of the spinal cord, the brain stem, and the cranial nerve nuclei according to René Bourdiol.[7]
c Auricular representation of the brain stem according to René Bourdiol.[7]
d Extrapyramidal motor areas according to René Bourdiol.[7]

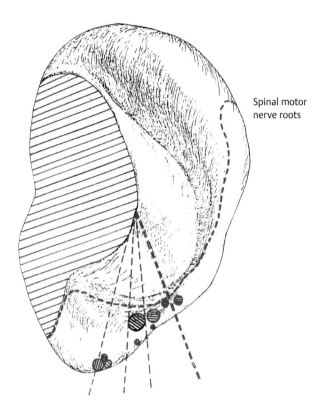

Spinal motor nerve roots

b

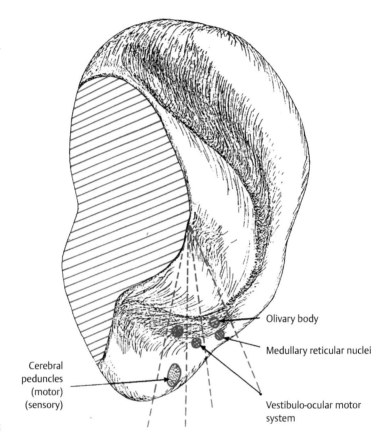

Olivary body

Medullary reticular nuclei

Cerebral peduncles (motor) (sensory)

Vestibulo-ocular motor system

c

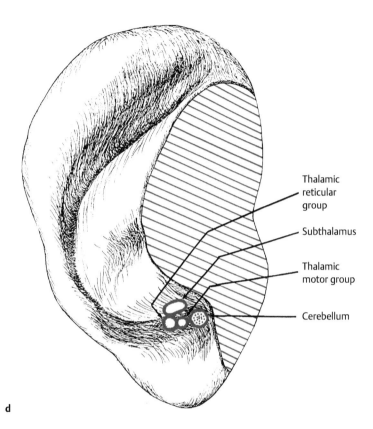

Thalamic reticular group

Subthalamus

Thalamic motor group

Cerebellum

d

Important Points on the Posterior Surface

The points on the anterior surface of the ear are largely related to sensory functions whereas those on the posterior surface are principally concerned with motor functions. For example:

- **Eye:** Convergence problems, strabismus
- **Maxilla:** Temporomandibular joint disorders
- **Shoulders:** Pectoral girdle imbalance
- **Pelvis:** Tilted pelvis
- **Rectum:** Incontinence
- **Urinary bladder:** Incontinence
- **Stomach:** Cramps

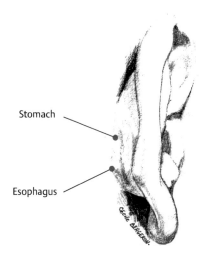

Stomach

Esophagus

a

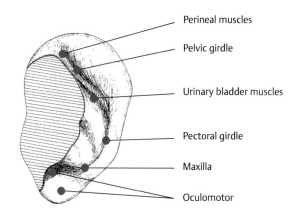

Perineal muscles

Pelvic girdle

Urinary bladder muscles

Pectoral girdle

Maxilla

Oculomotor

b

Fig. 49a, b Points for motor function.

Geometric Relationships

The pathologic points discovered on the ear often form patterns and are sometimes organized in geometrical lines.

- A radius vector passing through a somatic point defines a border point (on the rim of the helix), which has an enhanced effect on this somatic point. *A radius vector is a virtual line which originates at point zero and passes through the location of a vertebra or an organ.*
- A border point affects all the points located along its radius vector.
- The angle made by the lines linking the points on the ear is frequently 30°.
- Any point linked to a border point by a line forming an angle of 30° affects the border point and its own radius vector.
- A protractor should be used to measure the angles between the lines connecting the points.

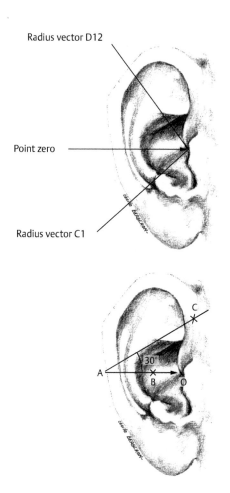

Fig. 50a, b Point A has an effect on point B because point B is located on point A's radius vector. Point C has an effect on both points A and B because the angle OAC = 30°.

Treatment of Aligned Points

The harmonic system:
It is not unusual to discover aligned points located on a radius vector passing through point zero. This is a harmonic system, and in such a case it is sufficient to treat a single point: the external point which is located at the helix on the same radius.

This system is often used in the intercostal zone.

The nonharmonic system:
In this situation, three or more points are aligned, but they do not create a vector passing through point zero. A protractor is used to locate a point at the intersection of the lines from which 30° angles may be made with these points. One line must pass through point zero. When needled, this derived point will deactivate the other points. This is called a **secondary harmonic point**.

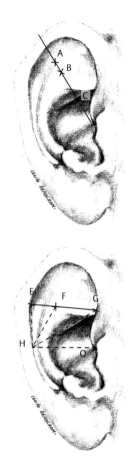

Fig. 51a, b

a **Harmonic system**. If the three points A, B, and C are in alignment, and if they are on a radius vector passing through point zero, the single point D located on the helix rim and on the radius vector may be treated by itself.

b **Nonharmonic system**. If the three points, E, F, and G are aligned, but they are not situated on a radius vector, another point H from which 30° angles may be made should be located. This is the single point which may be treated by itself.

Prioritizing the Points

Prioritization according to the points' position on the auricle:
The choice of points to treat is crucial. The order in which the points should be treated is of equal importance. Therapeutic results vary according to the order in which the points are treated.

Two simple rules apply in 90% of the situations that will be encountered:
- **The points should be needled in the following order:**
  - Points in the area innervated by the superficial cervical plexus
  - Points in the area innervated by the trigeminal nerve (CN V)
  - Points in the area innervated by the vagus nerve (CN X).
- **In any given area, the points furthest from point zero should be treated first.**

Prioritization according the points' symptomatology:
If two points are located symmetrically on each ear, or two points are very close to one another, one may choose:
- The most sensitive point, if found using the pressure probe method, or
- The point with the lowest resistance, if found using an electrodetector.

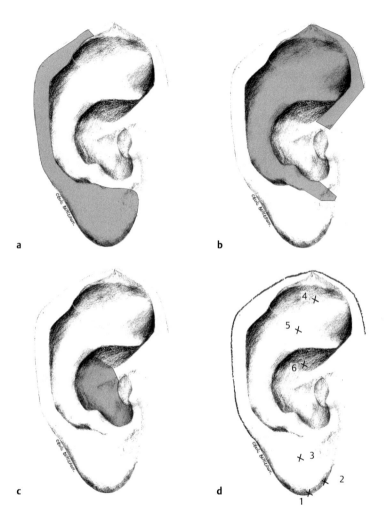

Fig. 52a–d
a Innervation by the superficial cervical plexus.
b Innervation by cranial nerve V (trigeminal nerve).
c Innervation by cranial nerve X (vagus nerve).
d Example: points 1–6 should be needled in the order shown above.

Paul Nogier's Phase Theory

The phase theory was proposed by Paul Nogier in the early 1980s. This theory presents the following observation:

When a point on the ear is needled, one primary and two secondary effects are frequently observed. The primary effect may be ectodermic, mesodermic, or endodermic.

- If the primary effect of needling the point is **ectodermic**, the secondary effects will be mesodermic and endodermic.
- If the primary effect is **mesodermic**, then the secondary effects will be ectodermic and endodermic.
- If the primary effect is **endodermic**, then the secondary effects will be ectodermic and mesodermic.

Paul Nogier therefore described three regions on the ear: T1, T2, and T3; he also described three tissue layers: superficial, middle, and deep. When a needle is inserted into the ear it passes through the three tissue layers. This accounts for three distinct effects caused by the needle.

In Paul Nogier's phase theory, there are three different somatotopes projected onto each one of these tissue layers:

- The somatotope of an **inverted fetus**.
- The somatotope of a **recumbent adult**.
- The somatotope of a **standing adult**.

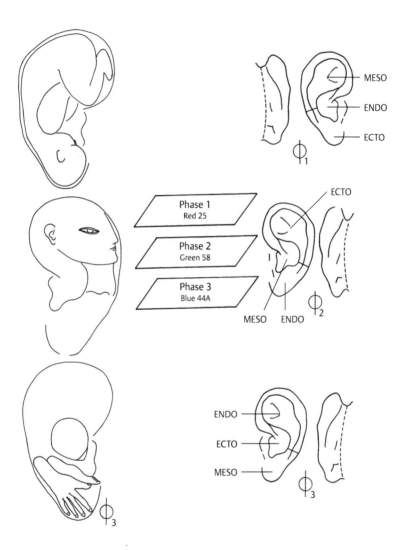

Fig. 53 According to Paul Nogier three somatotopes are superimposed on the ear.

A Contemporary Perspective on the Phases and Their Clinical Use Today

A current explanation of the phases:

When Paul Nogier published his phase theory, the structure of the ear points was not really known. Today we know about the neurovascular complexes, and it is hard to defend the existence of three superimposed somatotopes. On the other hand, it is possible that when a point on the ear is stimulated, that stimulus could be integrated on several levels by the nervous system. David Alimi,[12] University of Paris, thinks that these levels of integration could be:

- Medullary
- Thalamic
- Cortical

We will refer to these levels of integration as phases 1, 2, and 3.

At the international symposium in Puerto Rico in 2002 a working group comprising Drs. John Ackerman, Bryan Franck, Michel Marignan, and Raphael Nogier proposed an official definition of the phases:

"The phases are transient neurological representations of the body on the ear. They are the result of an integrative cerebral response to data, including environmental inputs, which result in physiological or pathological conditions."

Utilizing the phases:

The phase 1 depicted in all ear charts is the one used in most of the cases. When the clinical response is inadequate, one must then search for points in the other phases. These points can be identified using the method of electrodetection and are treated with needles.

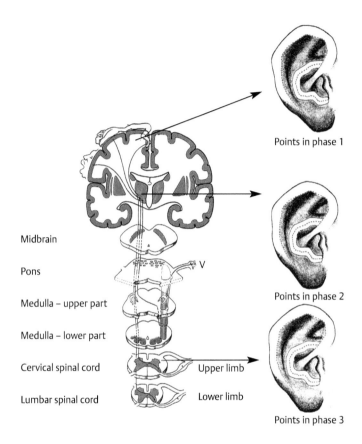

Points in phase 1

Midbrain

Pons

Medulla – upper part

Medulla – lower part

Cervical spinal cord

Lumbar spinal cord

V

Upper limb

Lower limb

Points in phase 2

Points in phase 3

Fig. 54 The effects of the phase points will depend on their level of interpretation by the nervous system:
Cortical interpretation = phase 1
Thalamic interpretation = phase 2
Medullary interpretation = phase 3

Phase 1

- This phase is observed in about 90% of cases.
- It is the most studied and best known of the phases.
- Paul Nogier described it as the metabolic tissue phase.

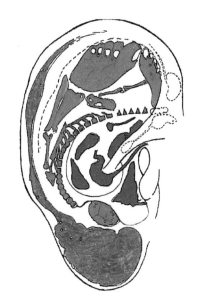

a

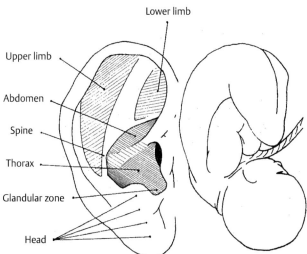

b

Fig. 55 a, b
a Auricular locations (Paul Nogier, 1977).
b The auricle and the corresponding fetal image (Paul Nogier, 1969).

■ *Phase 2*

According to Paul Nogier, this phase corresponds to the nerve-related aspect of the location.

Fig. 56a, b Endoderm: phase 2 according to Paul Nogier. ▶

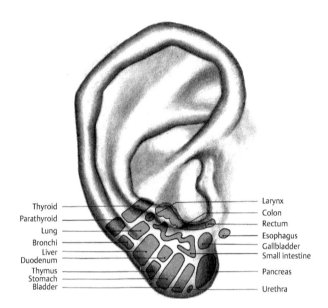

Thyroid
Parathyroid
Lung
Bronchi
Liver
Duodenum
Thymus
Stomach
Bladder

Larynx
Colon
Rectum
Esophagus
Gallbladder
Small intestine
Pancreas
Urethra

a

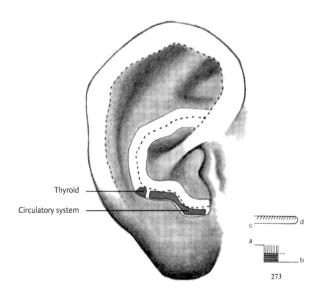

Thyroid
Circulatory system

c ———— d
a ———— b

273

b

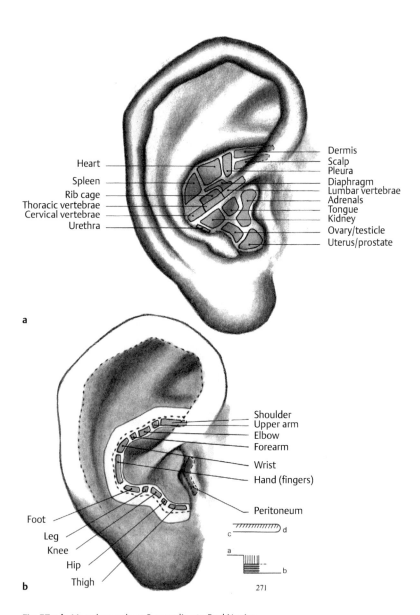

Fig. 57a, b Mesoderm: phase 2 according to Paul Nogier.

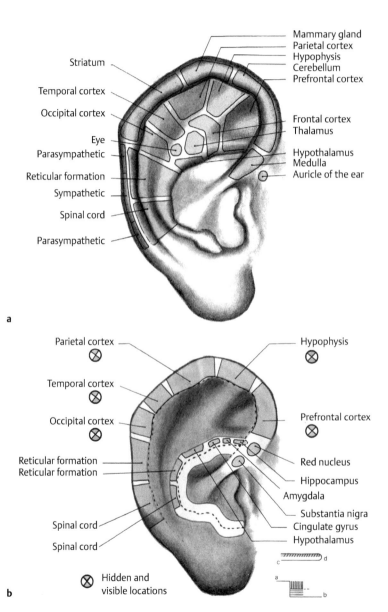

Fig. 58a, b Ectoderm: phase 2 according to Paul Nogier.

■ *Phase 3*

"This phase is essentially linked to the individual's energetic conformation." (Paul Nogier)

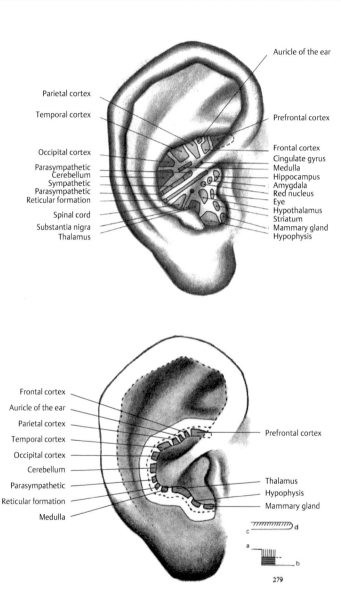

Fig. 59a, b Ectoderm: phase 3 according to Paul Nogier.

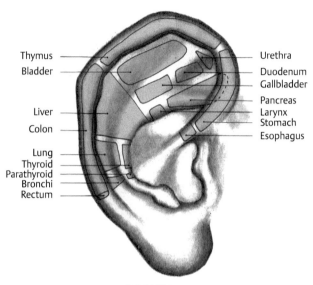

Thymus
Bladder
Liver
Colon
Lung
Thyroid
Parathyroid
Bronchi
Rectum

Urethra
Duodenum
Gallbladder
Pancreas
Larynx
Stomach
Esophagus

ENDODERM - φ 3

a

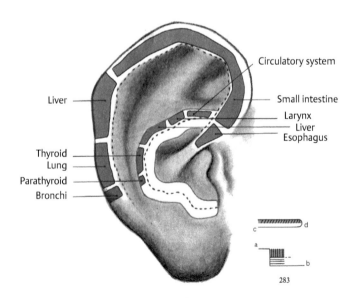

Liver

Thyroid
Lung
Parathyroid
Bronchi

Circulatory system
Small intestine
Larynx
Liver
Esophagus

283

b

Fig. 60a, b Endoderm: phase 3 according to Paul Nogier.

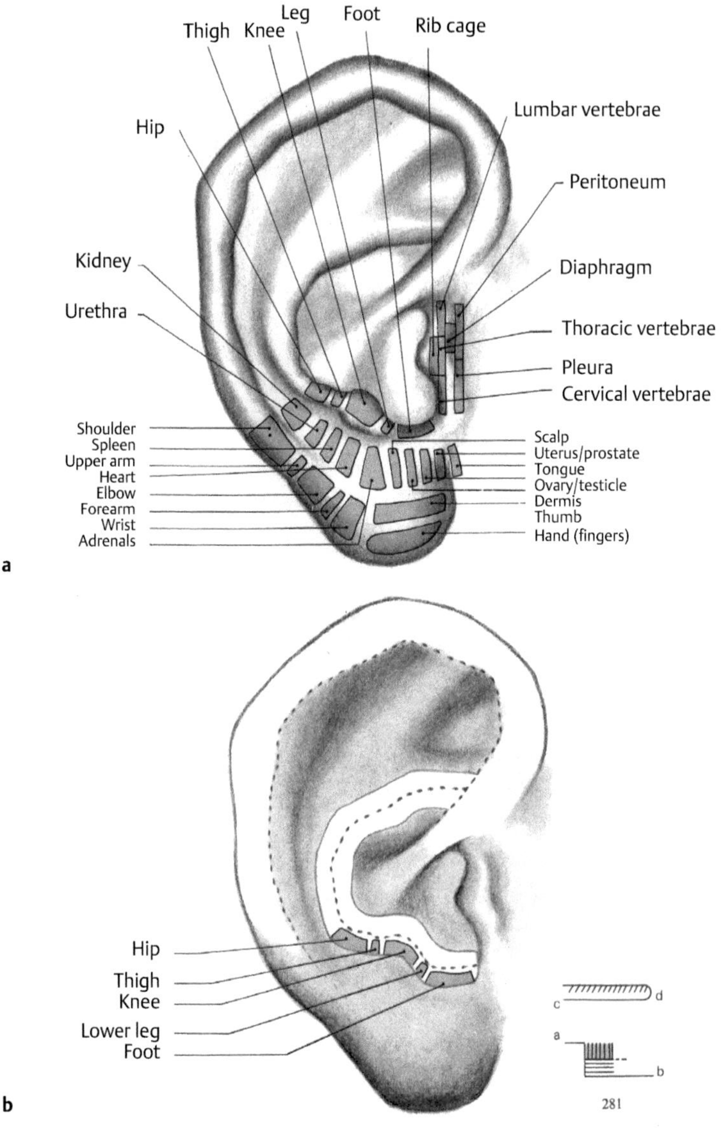

Fig. 61a, b Mesoderm: phase 3 according to Paul Nogier.

The Auricular-Cardiac Reflex (ACR), Also Known as Vascular Autonomic Signal (VAS)

In 1968 Paul Nogier made a chance discovery. While he was stimulating certain points of the ear, he felt a change in the patient's radial pulse. Sometimes the pulse became stronger, at other times it became weaker. He thought that there was a correlation between auricular stimulation and cardiac activity. He named this phenomenon auricular-cardiac reflex (ACR).

Eventually, Paul Nogier came to realize that any stimulation of the skin would bring about a vascular reaction. At Pierre Magnin's suggestion, the term ACR was replaced by vascular autonomic signal (VAS).

- This arterial phenomenon has also subsequently been called "Nogier's arterial reflex."
- Indeed, ACR, VAS, and Nogier's arterial reflex refer to the same phenomenon.
- **The ACR is a sign of the organism's adaptation to pain, cutaneous stimulation, emotion, or any abnormal situation.**
- If the technique of taking the pulse is mastered, the ACR enables one to evaluate the organism's adaptive capacity.
- The ACR has been the subject of much research. However, so far no procedure enables completely reliable recording of this phenomenon.

Fig. 62a, b ▶
a Method of taking the pulse to check for the auricular-cardiac reflex (ACR).
b The organism responds to external stimuli with an involuntary vascular reaction.

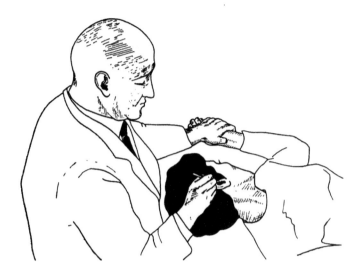

a

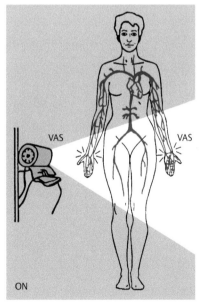

b

How to Experience the Vascular Autonomic Signal

Learning to sense the VAS is quite difficult. It requires patience and a long apprenticeship to master the phenomenon. The best way to train oneself is by taking the radial pulse of all of one's patients while stimulating some location of their skin with a bright light or physical pressure. Alternatively, simply create a stress with an unexpected sound like that of a falling object.

The VAS is an arterial reaction which is felt in the muscular tone of the (arterial) wall. It is not a matter of cardiac rhythm, which remains unchanged. The VAS manifests itself in the following ways:

- The pulse may become fuller, stronger.
- The pulse may become weaker, fainter.

The VAS response is immediate, as rapid as the pupillary retraction when the eye is exposed to a flash of light. It may last for one, two, or, most often, three beats. More than three beats generally indicates a pathologic condition.

The best way to learn this phenomenon is to build up experience by trying to sense the VAS in all of one's patients.

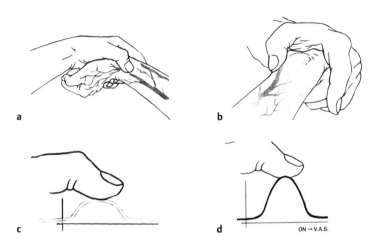

Fig. 63a–d

a The practitioner's thumb pressure on the patient's radial artery should be gentle.

b The practitioner's thumb should be placed lightly on the lateral side of the patient's radial artery.

c Visual representation of the pulse without the VAS.

d Visual representation of the pulse with the VAS in evidence.

Cutaneous Photoperception

Cutaneous photoperception is a phenomenon which was described following the discovery of the ACR. A bright light projected onto the skin of a "blind" mammal provokes an arterial reaction.

Numerous experiments performed at the Institut National des Sciences Appli-quées de Lyon (INSA, Lyon), particularly by Professor Roger Santini, clearly de-monstrated that a rabbit differentiates biologically between a pulsed and a con-tinuous light even if this light does not affect its eyes. The levels of dopamine, epinephrine, and norepinephrine were altered when a rabbit's back was exposed to a discontinous light stimulus.

It seems that the skin of mammals is not just a barrier between the external and internal environments, but it also functions as a site of communication between the two.

In fact, the skin seems to act as a vast electromagnetic information receiver.
This information almost certainly acts to stimulate and regulate the secretion of chemical neuromodulators.

The phenomenon of cutaneous photoperception integrates the concept of acupunc-ture points and auriculotherapy points. These points are, first and foremost, in-volved in this phenomenon. They can thus be studied by the physician as they take the radial pulse while researching VAS phenomena.

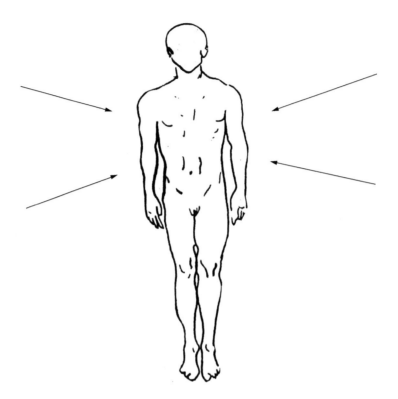

Fig. 64 The skin "photoperceives". We are immersed constantly in an electromagnetic sea. Using the skin as a receiver, electromagnetic waves stimulate, regulate, and restore some of the functions of an organism.

Cutaneous Photoperception and Ear Points

Normal physiological states:
In the resting state and in normal health it appears that the auricles of the ear have photoperceptive capacity only at the base frequencies. If a point of light is projected onto the skin of the auricle there is no VAS response. On the other hand, light stimulation of the rest of the body does trigger a VAS reaction.

Pathology:
In pathologic states, certain points on the ear become sensitive to light, and a point of light projected onto the ear triggers a VAS response.

Auriculotherapy treatment consists in "deactivating" the auricular points.

To sum up:
The skin of mammals is endowed with *photoperception*, the role of which is to *stimulate*, *regulate*, and *repair* the system. If an organism is in good health, the faculty of photoperception is active on its entire skin except on the skin of the ears. However, in the event of disease, the ear points will show active photoperception in order to return the system to homeostasis.

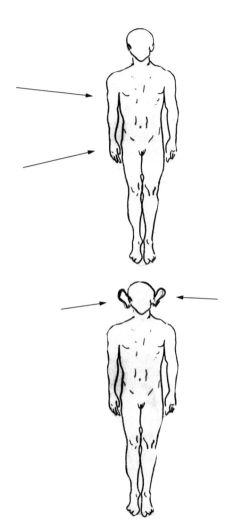

Fig. 65a, b
a In normal physiologic states, there is no auricular photoperception.
b Auricular photoperception is active only in pathologic conditions.

The Nogier Frequencies

In 1977 Paul Nogier established that:
- In terms of photoperception, the skin of the body can be divided into seven zones (See **Fig. 66a**)
- Regarding photoperception, the skin of the ear can similarly be divided into seven different zones (See **Fig. 66b**)
- Each zone on the body and the ear has a photoperceptive faculty specific to itself and "photoperceives" seven distinct frequencies.
- These seven frequencies are referred to as A, B, C, D, E, F, and G. They are known as "Nogier frequencies."
- Besides reacting to their base frequency, any pathologic point on the ear will react to one or more of the other Nogier frequencies.
- The Nogier frequencies induce specific biological effects: Frequency A has an anti-inflammatory effect, frequency B affects circulation, and so on.
- In normal physiological states photoperception is standardized at the frequencies shown on the following diagram. In pathological states changes are observed in cutaneous photoperception.

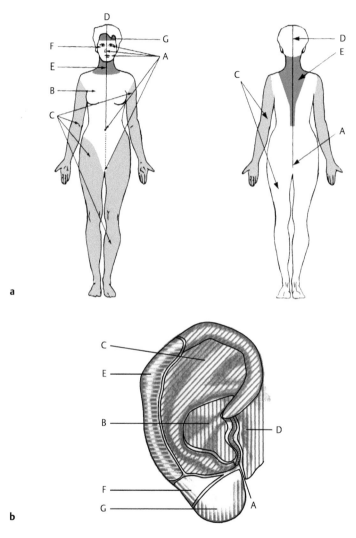

Fig. 66a, b
a The seven zones on the body.
b The seven zones on the ear.

■ *Frequency A*

2.28 Hertz

Color: orange, Kodak Wratten no. 21

Sites of photoperception:
- Auricular meatus
- Eyes
- Nostrils
- Mouth
- Umbilicus
- Urinary meatus
- Vagina
- Rectum

Effects of frequency A:
- Stimulation of cellular functions
- Anti-inflammatory
- Anti-edema

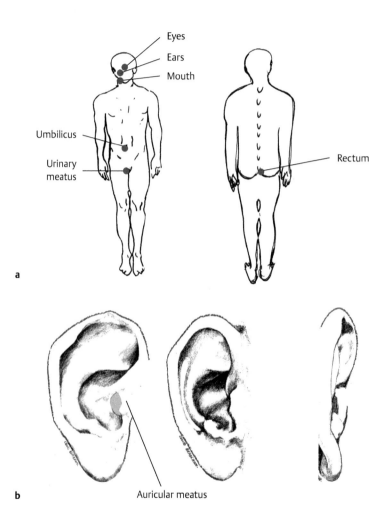

Fig. 67a, b Frequency A

■ *Frequency B*

4.56 Hertz

Color: red, Kodak Wratten no. 25

Sites of photoperception:
- On the body:
  - Anterior surface of the thorax and abdomen
- On the ear:
  - The concha

Effects of frequency B:
- Stimulation of digestive functions
- Stimulation of intercellular communication
- Stimulation of cellular cohesion as well as intercellular coherence
- Stimulation of immune functions: self, nonself recognition
- Antiallergy

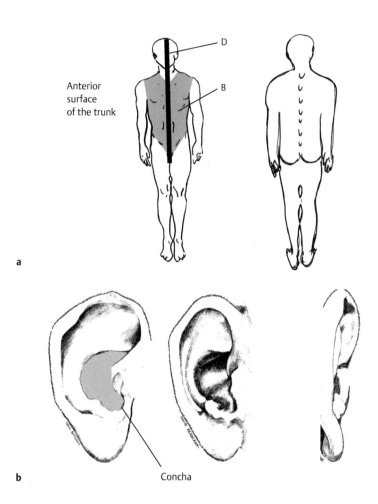

Anterior
surface
of the trunk

D

B

a

Concha

b

Fig. 68a, b Frequency B

▬ *Frequency C*

9.12 Hertz

Color: yellow, Kodak Wratten no. 3

Sites of photoperception:
- On the body:
  - Upper and lower limbs from proximal to distal extremities
- On the ear:
  - Antihelix
  - Helix (ascending branch, knee, and body)

Effects of frequency C:
- functions related to muscle contraction
- Stimulation of muscle agonist–antagonist relationships
- Stimulation of regulation of dopamine secretion

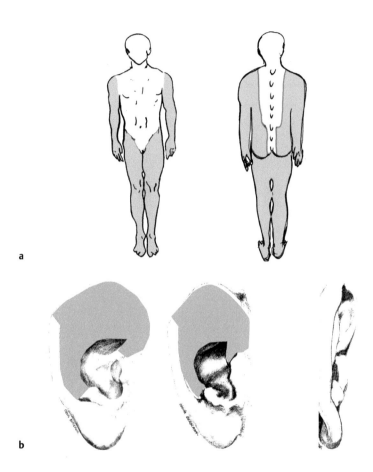

a

b

Fig. 69a, b Frequency C

■ *Frequency D*

18.25 Hertz

Color: red, Kodak Wratten no. 24

Sites of photoperception:
- On the body:
  - The sagittal line, on average 5 cm wide, beginning at the anus, then ascending along the vertebrae and passing over the top of the cranium to descend on the surface of the thorax and the abdomen, terminating at the urinary meatus
- On the ear:
  - The pretragal zone

Effects of frequency D:
Frequency D acts chiefly on functions related to spatial symmetry.

The property of symmetry is clearly a function of the nervous system. Unfortunately, this relationship has been overlooked in the past. From the moment that it starts to move, a living organism spontaneously creates an axis of symmetry. The organism must then learn to move its body parts about this axis in a coordinated manner to be able to move effectively. The nervous system has been organized to facilitate this phenomenon. Every evolved organism that translocates itself embodies a double system. The brain is divided into two hemispheres, each side controlling one half of the body. The two hemispheres are linked by interhemispheric nerve fibers.

Frequency D acts on these interhemispheric fibers and on functions related to symmetry:
- Motor functions
- Gait
- Posture

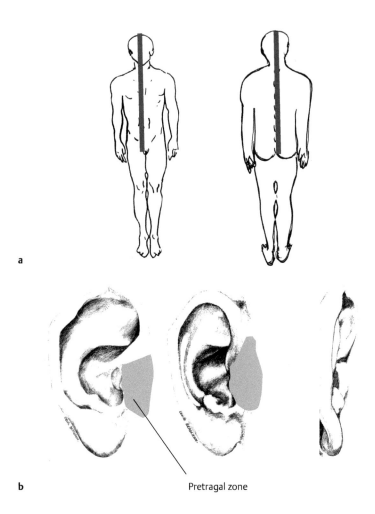

a

b

Pretragal zone

Fig. 70a, b Regularization of the autonomic system.

■ *Frequency E*

36.5 Hertz

Color: Blue, Kodak Wratten no. 44

Sites of photoperception:
- On the body:
  - Anterior and posterior surfaces of the neck
  - On the back over the spinal column
- On the ear:
  - Tail of the helix

Effects of frequency E:
- Stimulation of the spinal column
- Analgesia

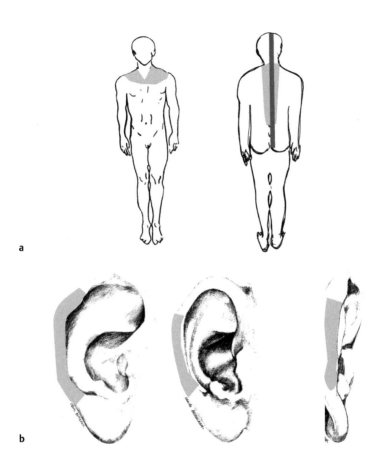

a

b

Fig. 71a, b Frequency E

■ *Frequency F*

73 Hertz

Color: violet, Kodak Wratten no.78

Sites of photoperception:
- On the body:
    - The face and the temporal region
- On the ear:
    - The lower region of the isthmus of the auricle where it encroaches on the lobe, but does not reach the tip. It proceeds along the foot of the concha, emerging on the posterior external surface

Effects of frequency F:
- Stimulation of the central grey nuclei
- Therapeutic effects:
    - Stimulation of growth hormone secretion
    - Healing: wounds, ulcers, bone fractures
    - Antidepressive
    - Regulation of hypothalamus
    - Appetite regulation

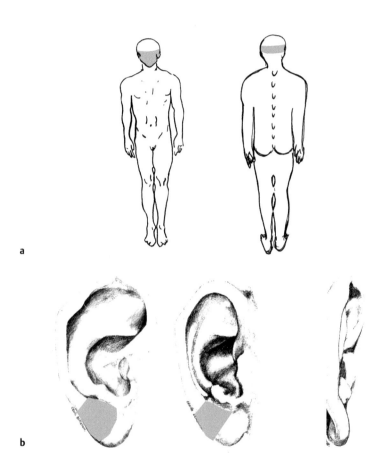

a

b

Fig. 72a, b Frequency F

■ *Frequency G*

146 Hertz

Color: rose, Kodak Wratten no. 31

Sites of photoperception:
- On the body:
  - Skull
  - Forehead
  - Nostrils
- On the ear:
  - Anterior region of the lobe

The effects of frequency G:
- Stimulation of the cerebral cortex

Clinical applications:
- Auxiliary point for epilepsy
- Psychosomatic disorders
- Treatment of chronic pain

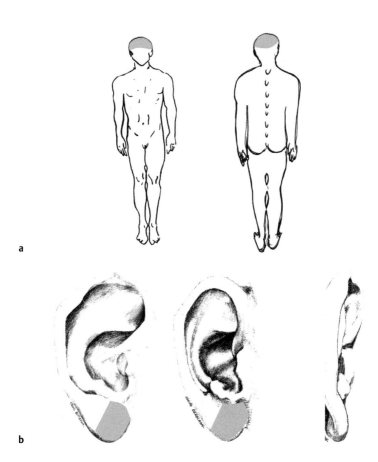

a

b

Fig. 73a, b Frequency G

How to Select Equipment for Studying the Nogier Frequencies and Treating Ear Points

Many different devices are available for studying photoperception at the Nogier frequencies. Some use red light emitting diodes (LEDs), others work with infrared light, and still others work with a white light. Some of the devices operate with laser light.

Some guidelines should be observed when using these devices:

- Ensure that the frequencies offered are those specified by Paul Nogier.
- Select a device that operates preferentially in the infrared range. All the clinical studies conducted on the Nogier frequencies have been carried out with infrared rays. Furthermore, the infrared light rays are not impeded by hemoglobin in the blood, thus permitting deeper penetration.
- For diagnostic use, avoid purchasing a device that is too powerful or that is laser operated. These types of device will treat the points while they are being used for diagnosis, thus interfering with the examination and confounding the findings.
- Some manufacturers are offering devices with the fundamental frequencies and also with the option of varying them by plus or minus 30% in relation to the fundamental frequencies. This could be useful since these variable frequencies have a specific field of application in auriculotherapy.

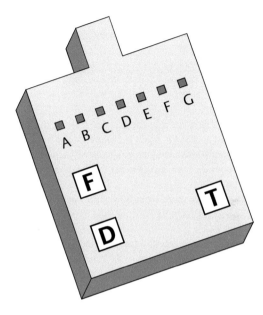

Fig. 74 Illustration of a generic device for measuring Nogier frequencies.
D = detection
T = treatment
F = frequencies

The Study of Ear Points by their Frequencies

Any auricular point in a pathologic state, detectable by pressure-induced pain or by an electrosensor can be analyzed and treated by using the Nogier frequencies.

Point analysis:
- Besides reacting to their base frequency, as described in the preceding text, any pathologic point on the ear will react to one or more of the other Nogier frequencies. To identify these frequencies, take the patient's radial pulse and check for VAS phenomena while projecting the frequencies (A, B, C, D, E, F, and G) onto the ear points one by one.
- When the **pulse becomes more forceful** while a particular frequency is being projected onto a point, that point is considered to be reactive to that frequency.
- When a **point on the ear reacts to a frequency other than that of the zone to which it belongs,** the frequency is considered to be parasitic.
- The **point is treated** with either the base frequency of the point or with the base frequency plus the parasitic frequency. For the treatment the frequencies are applied at higher power than those used for detection.
- **The duration of point treatment** with the frequency is variable, averaging about 30 seconds.
- Several **different points can be treated** with the frequencies during the same session.

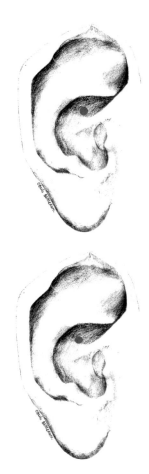

Fig. 75a, b
a This point in the concha reacts primarily to the B frequency.
b If the same point reacts to other frequencies (such as A, D, and F, for instance), the point should be treated with these frequencies.

The Electromagnetic Signature of a Lesion

The study of parasitic frequencies enables us to define a lesion of the organism and to study its electromagnetic characteristics. We call this an electromagnetic signature.

For example:
Mr. Dupont has come to the clinic with shoulder pain. With a frequency-triggered infrared beam we can ascertain whether the projection of any of the different frequencies onto the shoulder initiates a VAS response. Each frequency should be tested. Using this system a lesion can be identified. For example, if the projection of frequencies A, B, F, and G trigger a VAS reaction, we would say that the electromagnetic signature of Mr. Dupont's shoulder lesion is: A, B, F, G. In this case all the frequencies found are parasitic since the shoulder reacts normally only to frequency C.

The electromagnetic signature of a lesion is invaluable for finding an active point on the ear. The auricular point most effective relative to the shoulder pain shares the same electromagnetic characteristics—in this case, frequencies A, B, F, and G. We must therefore search for this point on the ear using an infrared frequency generator. Once found, this point should be needled.

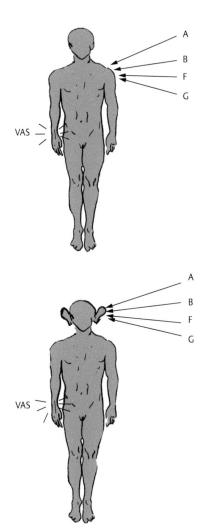

Fig. 76a, b

a In a case of pathology, first the VAS is utilized to search for photoreactive frequencies related to the lesion (e.g., shoulder pain).

b Second, a point on the ear with the same frequency characteristics is sought using the VAS reflex. This point should be needled.

The Treatment of Peripheral Neuropathies

The treatment of neuropathies with auricular techniques requires expertise in reading the VAS.

Neuropathies generally originate from metabolic diseases (e.g., diabetes) or autotoxicity (e.g., alcoholism). They manifest as highly disabling conditions, sometimes with extreme sensitivity of the extremities. Conventional therapies are limited and the results from their use are often disappointing. Unfortunately, neuroleptic drugs are neither well tolerated nor very effective.

Auricular treatment of neuropathies is based on the ability to work with the parasitic frequencies.

Treatment:

For example, in a case of diabetic neuropathy of the lower limbs:

1. **Determine the electromagnetic signature of the affected areas**. We can identify the parasitic frequencies with an infrared frequency generator.
2. **Search for a point on one of the ears** with the same signature. To accomplish this the patient's pulse is taken while the frequencies are projected onto each ear.
3. The **point with the same signature is needled**.
4. **Check the frequency of the affected areas**. If the auricular point that has been identified is the right one, the affected limb should respond only to its specific frequency, in this case frequency C.

Fig. 77a, b Treating neuropathies of the lower limbs. For example: ▶
a 1. Use the VAS to find reactive frequencies on the skin of the lower limbs, e.g., A, B, E, F, G.
b 2. Search on the ear for one or more points reactive to these same frequencies, i.e., A, B, E, F, G.
   3. This (or these) point(s) may be needled.
   4. Treatment sessions should be repeated monthly.

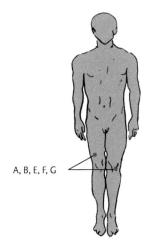

A, B, E, F, G

a

A, B, E, F, G

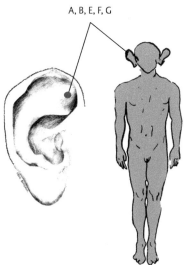

b

The Treatment of Fibromyalgia

Fibromyalgia is a commonly seen disease, characterized by musculoskeletal pain with readily occurring stiffness and fatigue. It primarily affects women between 25 and 45 years of age. The etiology and pathogenesis of this disorder are unknown.

Treatment:
- **Needles should not be used** in the treatment of fibromyalgia, since their use will exacerbate the symptoms of fatigue and pain. Treatment should be performed solely by infrared frequencies on the ear.
- The **points should be selected from those located on the concha**. These points can usually be identified by electrodetection and should be treated with infrared light at frequency B.
- These **points should be treated every 15 days** for about 6 months. After this the frequency of treatment sessions will vary according to the needs of the individual.

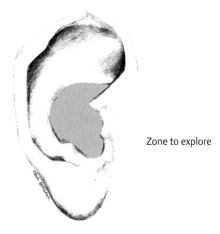

Zone to explore

Fig. 78 The treatment of fibromyalgia. Zone to explore: The pathologic points on the concha must be located. This can be accomplished with an electrodetector. The points thus identified should be treated with frequency B.

The Treatment of Depressive Disorder

Depressive disorder is becoming more and more common. Diagnosis is made on the basis of at least five of the following **symptoms** being present over a period of 2 weeks:
- Sadness
- Indifference to or loss of pleasure in normally enjoyed activities
- Insomnia or hypersomnia
- Significant weight gain or loss
- Lethargy or agitation
- Fatigue
- Feelings of guilt or worthlessness
- Difficulty in concentrating or making decisions
- Thoughts of death or suicide

Auriculotherapy is a very effective treatment for clinical depression when the disorder is of recent onset and is reactive.

Treatment:
The **essential points** to check are:
- Point O′, left and right
- Points on the anterior region of the lobe corresponding to the prefrontal cortex
- Right and left hypothalamus points
- Right and left hypophysis points
- Superior and inferior concha points on the right and left sides

These points can be treated regularly with needles and also by infrared light, mainly at their base frequencies.

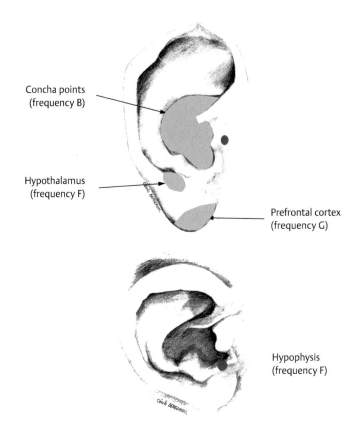

Concha points
(frequency B)

Hypothalamus
(frequency F)

Prefrontal cortex
(frequency G)

a

Hypophysis
(frequency F)

b

Fig. 79a, b The treatment of clinical depression.

Appendix

■ *About the Author*

Son of the famous Paul Nogier, the founder of auriculotherapy, Raphael Nogier became a specialist in this area of treatment early on when working on research together with his father. Following his father's death, Raphael Nogier further developed his father's work. As a practicing physician, he has set new standards in auriculotherapy.

Raphael Nogier runs his medical practice in Lyon, France, where he practices his form of therapy. He is the author of numerous studies and books. Since 1977 he has taught auriculotherapy at many different schools in many countries throughout the world.

Raphael Nogier currently works with the "Groupe Lyonnais d'Etudes Médicales" (Medical Study Group of Lyon) and organizes the "Journées Médicales de Septembre" (Medical Days in September). For more information please see www .nogier.info.

Since 1989, he has acted as rapporteur in the World Health Organization's Scientific Group on International Acupuncture Nomenclature. He was president of the working group on the standardization of the nomenclature of the ear acupuncture points in Lyon 1990.

■ Auriculotherapy

Auriculotherapy is a method of treatment that utilizes the reflexive properties of the auricle of the ear. It was discovered by Paul Nogier in Lyon, France, in 1951. Since then it has been the subject of numerous neurophysiological studies.

In 1990 a working group convened by the World Health Organization (WHO) standardized the nomenclature of 43 auricular points.

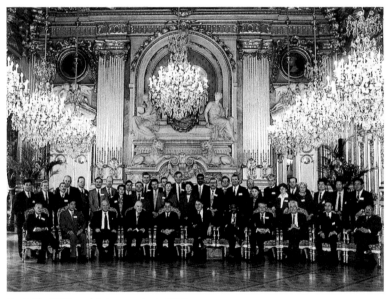

Fig. 1 The WHO working group—Lyon, 1990

Dr Hiroshi Nakajima
Director General, World Health Organization

"Mr. Chairman, Dr. Paul Nogier, distinguished members of the Working Group, ladies and gentlemen,

... As you know, the efforts of the World Health Organization in standardizing auricular acupuncture points began as part of the deliberations of the third Working Group on the Standardization of Acupuncture Nomenclature, which met in Seoul in 1987. Auricular acupuncture is probably the most developed, and the best documented scientifically, of all the microsystems of acupuncture; it is also the most practical and widely used. Ear acupuncture is mentioned now and then in some Chinese acupuncture classics, but no extensive or in-depth deliberations are recorded. Obviously, it was not considered to be part of the main body of classical acupuncture. Unlike classical acupuncture, which is almost entirely derived from ancient China, auricular acupuncture is, to a large extent, a more recent development that has received considerable contributions from the West.

This is why we are privileged to have with us today Dr. Paul Nogier. As you know, Dr. Nogier has devoted a considerable part of his career to the study and use of acupuncture in Europe, and especially to the theory and clinical application of auricular therapy.

His suggestion that there is a relationship between the fetal position and the adult ear contributed to the development of auricular acupuncture and, later, auricular medicine.

Essentially on the basis of his work, ear charts have been published in many countries throughout the world. While they show varying degrees of difference, they all have as their basis the same fetal configuration described by Dr. Nogier.

It is WHO's intention to promote and recommend for international use a complete standardized auricular acupuncture nomenclature. We expect that this will facilitate serious research into auricular therapy by allowing for replication of scientific studies and for comparability of research results.

In closing, may I take this opportunity to acknowledge with great pleasure the debt of honor that modern medicine owes to Dr. Paul Nogier, a distinguished son of Lyon.

Thank you very much."

Lyon, France, 1990

▬ *Glossary*

ACR
Auricular-cardiac reflex (*see* (→) VAS).

Amygdala
A group of almond-shaped nuclei located beneath the anterior part of the temporal lobe, comprising an important part of the (→) limbic system. The amygdala integrates sensory and visceral information with records of past evolutionary experience and communicates extensively with the forebrain, the (→) hypothalamus, and the brainstem. Its outputs stimulate the hypothalamus to release the neurotransmitters dopamine, norepinephrine, and epinephrine which activate the sympathetic nervous system.

Auriculomedicine
A field of medicine originated by Dr. Paul Nogier in the 1970s, based on his discovery of the photoperceptive properties of the skin, its sensitivity to specific frequencies of light at specific locations, and the possibility of exploiting these phenomena in the diagnosis and treatment of disease. *See* (→) Nogier frequencies.

Basal ganglia
The basal ganglia (or basal nuclei) are a group of nuclei in the brain interconnected with the (→) cerebral cortex, (→) the thalamus, and the brainstem. They are associated with motor control, cognition, emotions, and learning.

Cerebellum
The cerebellum integrates sensory information for postural balance, manages the coordination of skilled, voluntary movements, and regulates muscle tone. It also has a role in the focusing of attention and the processing of language, music, and other sensory stimuli.

It is located in the posterior part of the brain under the occipital lobe, and comprises about 10% of the brain's mass.

Cerebral cortex
The cerebral cortex has a key role in the processing of information related to memory, attention, sensory perception, perceptual awareness, thought, language, and consciousness. Planning, creativity, decision making, the initiation of voluntary actions, and self-consciousness occur in this area.

The cerebral cortex consists of the convoluted surface layer of the cerebral hemispheres of which two-thirds is folded into grooves (sulci). It is divided into sensory, motor, and association areas.

The cerebral cortex communicates with subcortical structures including the ($\rightarrow$) thalamus and ($\rightarrow$) basal ganglia, receiving sensory (except olfactory) information from them via the thalamus. However, as many as 99% of the connections (according to Braitenberg and Schüz 1991) are actually from one area of the cortex to another.

Cerebral peduncles
Comprising most of the midbrain, this area contains many nerve tracts conveying motor information to and from the brain to the rest of the body.

Cingulate gyrus
A gyrus (ridge) in the medial part of the brain. It partially wraps around the ($\rightarrow$) corpus callosum. It functions as an integral part of the ($\rightarrow$) limbic system, which is involved in the formation and processing of emotions, learning, and memory.

Corpus callosum
A wide, flat bundle of axons beneath the cortex connecting the left and right cerebral hemispheres, across which much of the interhemispheric communication in the brain is conducted.

Ectoblast
The outer germinal layer of an early embryo, consisting of undifferentiated cells destined to become the ($\rightarrow$) ectoderm.

Ectoderm
One of the three embryonic germ layers. The ectoderm develops into: the brain; skin; nails; the epithelium of the nose, mouth, and anal canal; the lens of the eye; the retina; and the nervous system.

Endoblast
The inner germinal layer of an early embryo, consisting of undifferentiated cells destined to become the ($\rightarrow$) endoderm.

Endoderm
One of the three embryonic germ layers. The endoderm forms: the skeletal muscle; the skeleton; the dermis of the skin; the crystal lens of the eye; connective tissue; the urogenital system; the heart; blood (lymph cells); and the spleen.

Frontal cortex
A cortical region of the frontal lobe, also termed prefrontal association cortex, this area influences personality and is associated with higher mental functions such as long-range planning, forming, and manipulating concepts and moral discrimination. *See also* (→) prefrontal cortex.

The frontal cortex has extensive neuronal input from centers in the brainstem and from the (→) limbic regions.

Harmonic system
Aligned reactive points located on a radius vector passing through (→) point zero. In such a case it is sufficient to treat a single point; the furthest out from point zero, to deactivate all the other related points.

Hippocampus
Located in the forebrain in the medial temporal lobe, the hippocampus is a crucial part of the (→) limbic system, functioning in parallel with the survival-related input–output processing functions of the (→) amygdala. It processes intellectual, emotional, and factual information, and mediates input from the sensory cortex to the (→) prefrontal cortex. It is believed to complement the amygdaloid complex's encoding of emotional memories stored in the cortex by consolidating experience and short-term memory into long-term memory.

Hypophysis
Also termed the pituitary gland, the hypophysis is located at the base of the brain and functionally connected to the (→) hypothalamus by the pituitary stalk, along which hypothalamic-releasing factors stimulate the release of pituitary hormones.

These hormones are involved in the regulation of growth, blood pressure, aspects of pregnancy and childbirth (including the stimulation of uterine contractions during labor), breast milk production, sexual function, the thyroid gland, water and osmolarity in the body, and food metabolism.

Disorders of the pituitary gland include acromegaly, growth hormone deficiency, and hypertension.

Hypothalamus

Responsible for the regulation of homeostatic functions such as temperature control, food intake, and fluid balance in the body, the hypothalamus links the nervous system to the endocrine system via the pituitary gland (*see* [→] Hypophysis). The hypothalamus is situated below and in front of the (→) thalamus, and is about the size of an almond.

It synthesizes and secretes neurohormones, which in turn inhibit or stimulate the secretion of the pituitary hormones that act directly on physiological functions.

Limbic system

A ring of cortex surrounding the (→) corpus callosum (an arch of transverse fibers connecting the right and left cerebral hemispheres) including the subcallosal and (→) cingulate gyri plus the parahippocampal gyrus. Its functions are concerned with the survival of the individual and the continuation of the species, including feeding and aggressive behaviors, emotional expression, and sexual response.

Locus niger

Also termed substantia nigra, the locus niger is a major part of the (→) basal ganglia system. It is composed of two distinct assemblies: one comprises elements of the core of the basal ganglia. The other, with its surrounding area is responsible for dopamine production in the brain and has a vital role in reward and addiction.

Location

The process of determining or marking the location or site of an organ, lesion, or disease on the auricle.

Master oscillation point

One of the auricular (→) master points, the oscillation point is located on the tragus, and treats problems of cerebral laterality by balancing left and right cerebral hemispheres. It appears to be the same, or close to the same location as Nogier's O'.

Master points

A group of points on the ear with generalized action, which can be combined for use in a wide variety of treatments.

They include:

- *Endocrine*: activates the entire hormonal system via the pituitary gland (*see* (→) Hypophysis).
- Stress control: activates the adrenal to buffer acute and chronic stress.

- *Tranquilizer*: regulates blood pressure, relieves. muscle tension, and has a general sedative effect.
- *Master cerebral*: treats chronic pain and psychosomatic disorders.
- (→) *Master oscillation*: treats problems of cerebral laterality by balancing left and right cerebral hemispheres.
- *Master sensorial*: helps to ensure accurate perception in the five senses.
- (→) *Point zero*: helps to enable physical homeostasis.
- *Shen men*: reduces anxiety and pain and raises the mood.
- *Sympathetic*: regulates blood circulation and the overall functioning of the autonomic nervous system.
- *Thalamus*: used for pain control.

Medulla
Also known as the medulla oblongata and the brainstem, the medulla is the lower part of the brain, adjoining and structurally continuous with the spinal cord below and the pons above. It relays nerve signals between the brain and spinal cord and regulates the autonomic nervous system's functions of respiration, blood pressure, swallowing, vomiting, and defecation.

Mesoblast
The middle germinal layer of an early embryo, consisting of undifferentiated cells destined to become the (→) mesoderm.

Mesoderm
One of the three embryonic germ layers. The mesoderm forms precursor tissues, which give rise to the muscles, and the circulatory and excretory systems of the body.

Nonharmonic system
In this situation, three or more points are aligned but do not create a vector passing through (→) point zero. A protractor is used to locate a point at the intersection of lines from which 30° angles may be made with these points and (→) point zero. When needled, this derived point will deactivate the other points. This is called a secondary harmonic point.

Neurovascular complex
Also termed neurovascular hemolymphatic complex, it has been identified as the basic histologic structure of acupuncture points on the body and the ear.

It consists of a lymphatic stem coupled to a large arteriole with one branch ascending vertically toward the epidermis and accompanied by a venule. Myelinated nerve fibers are intertwined with the blood and lymph vessels and netlike structures of unmyelinated nerve fibers surround the vessels. The whole structure is located in a vertical column of loose connective tissue that arises from the superficial fascia and is surrounded by thick, dense, partially insulating dermal connective tissue.

The surface of the skin above the neurovascular complexes has been measured to be consistently in the order of 1000 times more electrically conductive than the surrounding tissue.

Nogier frequencies
The cutaneous surface of the body and the ear can be divided into seven zones (A–G). When exposed to light flashing at one of seven specific frequencies, they have discrete biologic effects on the body due to the photoperceptive properties of the skin. The frequencies are standard in normal physiologic states but become atypical in pathologic situations. The vascular autonomic signal (VAS) is monitored to determine to which frequency (or frequencies) a zone is reactive.

The exploitation of these phenomena in diagnosis and treatment of pathology forms the basis of Nogier's ($\rightarrow$) auriculomedicine.

Nucleus
A term in neuroanatomy referring to a structure in the central nervous system composed primarily of neurons, which acts as a hub for signal routing in a neural subsystem.

Occipital cortex
The cortex of the occipital lobe, which is the visual processing region of the brain. It controls vision and color recognition, and plays a part in the sense of hearing.

Olivary body
About the size and shape of an olive and located on the brain stem, it is composed of two groups of nuclei. The upper ($\rightarrow$) nucleus is part of the auditory processing system and aids in the perception of sound.

The lower nuclei are mainly dedicated to cerebellar motor learning and motor function.

Parasympathetic
The parasympathetic nervous system (PNS) is part of the autonomic nervous system (ANS), which also includes the sympathetic nervous system (SNS) and the enteric (bowel-related) nervous system (ENS). The ANS forms part of the peripheral nervous system. The PNS is responsible for activities concerned with metabolic rest and regeneration. It complements and balances the activities of the SNS, which is responsible for activities related to immediate survival ("fight or flight") and typically involve the use of large amounts of physiologic resources.

Parietal cortex
The cortex of the parietal lobe in the brain, situated posterior to the frontal lobe and superior to the occipital lobe. It is concerned with integrating sensory information from various parts of the body and determining spatial sense and orientation.

Phase theory of Paul Nogier
The phase theory was proposed by Dr. Paul Nogier in about 1980. This theory proposes that when a point on the ear is needled, one primary and two secondary effects are frequently observed. The primary effect may be (→) ectodermic, (→) mesodermic, or (→) endodermic. Secondary effects will be related to the other two embryonic germ layers.

In 2002, Dr. Raphael Nogier was a member of a working group that issued the following official definition of the phases:

"The phases are transient neurological representations of the body on the ear. They are the result of an integrative cerebral response to data, including environmental inputs, which result in physiological or pathological conditions."

Photoperception
The sensitivity of the skin to light and its ability to transmit information coded in light vibrating at specific frequencies to the central nervous system.

Point zero
One of the auricular (→) master points. Point zero helps to enable physical homeostasis.

Prefrontal cortex
The anterior part of the frontal lobes of the brain. Its basic activity is believed to be the coordination of thoughts and actions in alignment with internal aims and objectives. The prefrontal cortex is associated with "executive functions" including long-term planning and drive, the capacity to recognize future consequences

resulting from present actions, to override and suppress inappropriate social responses, and discriminate between salient factors in things or events.

Radius vector
A radius vector is a virtual line which originates at (→) point zero and passes through the (→) location of a vertebra or an organ.

Red nucleus
A structure in the midbrain involved in upper body motor coordination (including arm swinging while walking) and crawling in babies.

Reticular formation
Part of the autonomic nervous system involved in the regulation of respiration, heart rate, and gastrointestinal activity. It modulates states of consciousness ranging from alertness to sleep, including fatigue and motivation, and is associated with the sensation of pain.

This formation is situated at the core of the brainstem and runs through the midbrain, pons, and medulla. It connects to areas in the (→) thalamus, (→) the hypothalamus and (→) cortex above, and the (→) cerebellum and sensory nerves below.

Somatotopy
Describes a constant spatial relationship between an area on the surface of the body and the central nervous system. For instance, points on the ear affecting organs, limbs or neural structures are represented in a corresponding spatial relationship in the brain.

Striatum (striate body)
Anatomically the caudate (→) nucleus and the putamen, the striatum is the major input relay of the (→) basal ganglia complex. It plays a part in executive function and is activated by stimuli associated with reward, punishment, or surprise in accord with the intensity and contextual relevance of the stimulus.

Associated pathologies include Parkinson disease, Huntington disease, dyskinesias, and possibly addiction disorders.

Subthalamus
Also termed prethalamus and ventral thalamus, it relays nerve impulses to the (→) striatum, the dorsal (→) thalamus, the (→) red nucleus, and the substantia nigra, but it does not communicate directly with the cortex. It receives inputs from the substantia nigra and the striatum.

Sympathetic
One of the auricular (→) master points, the sympathetic point regulates blood circulation and the overall functioning of the autonomic nervous system. Also, the name for a part of the autonomic nervous system. *See* (→) Parasympathetic.

Temporal cortex
The cortex of the temporal lobes, which are located on each side of the brain. The temporal cortex includes the primary auditory cortex and is involved in auditory processing as well as semantics, speech, and vision.

Thalamic reticular group
A group of nuclei forming part of the (→) subthalamus, which relay nerve impulses to the (→) striatum, the dorsal (→) thalamus, the (→) red nucleus, and the (→) substantia nigra. However, the thalamic reticular group does not communicate directly with the (→) cerebral cortex. It receives inputs from the substantia nigra and the (→) striatum.

Thalamus
This preprocesses and relays a wide variety of (→) subthalamic inputs to the (→) cerebral cortex. It has multiple connections both to and from the cerebral cortex potentially forming feedback loops, and may play a part in conscious awareness.

It has a major role in regulating states of consciousness ranging from deep sleep to alert wakefulness, including levels of arousal and activity.

Pathologically, damage resulting from cerebrovascular accidents (strokes) may result in contralateral paresthesias or numbness and emotional disturbances, a condition known as thalamic syndrome. Damage to the organ may also result in irreversible coma. *See also* (→) Master points.

VAS
The vascular autonomic signal, also formerly termed (→) ACR (auricular-cardiac reflex). A characteristic response found in the radial pulse to a variety of sensory inputs.

Vestibulo-ocular motor system
Part of the vestibulo-ocular reflex, it stabilizes visual images on the retina to compensate for head movement by moving the eyes in the opposite direction to the movement of the head.

References for Glossary

Braitenberg and Schüz ,1991
Cho ZH, Wong EK, Fallon J. Neuro-Acupuncture Q-Puncture Inc. Los Angeles, CA; 2001
Helms J M. Acupuncture Energetics—A clinical Approach for Physicians. Berkeley CA: Medical
Acupuncture Publishers; 1995
Sherwood L. Human Physiology From Cells to Systems, 2nd ed. Minneapolis: West Publishing
Company; 1995

▬ *Recommended Equipment and Supplies*

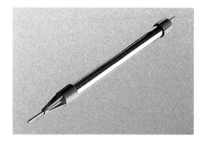

Pressure probe: 250 g pressure.
Essential for auriculotherapy.

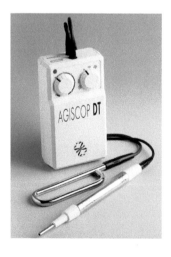

Point detector. Differential detection
capability is required for accurate readings.
The Agiscop DT is easy to use.

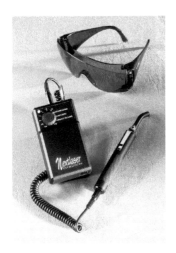

Laser. Infrared pulsed lasers must be used. The Nextlaser with a 904 nm diode is effective for treating auricular points.

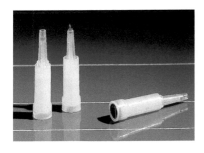

Intradermal (ASP semipermanent) needles.

Photos with kind permission of SEDATELEC, France.

References and Further Reading

■ *References*

1. Senelar R. Organisation du point d'acupuncture. Laboratoire d'Histologie-embryo-logie. Faculté de medicine de Montpellier. France, 1987
2. Terral C. Le point d'acupuncture. Conference, GLEM. Lyon, June 2007
3. Auziech O. Acupuncture et auriculothérapie. Essai d'analyse histologique de quelques structures cutanées impliquées dans ces deux techniques. Montpellier: Sauramps médical; 1985
4. Nogier R. Practical Introduction to Auriculomedicine [in French]. Heidelberg: Haug; 1993
5. Marignan M. Thermographie des points auriculaires. Lyon: Publication GLEM; 2000
6. Auziech, op. cit., 3
7. Bourdiol RJ. Eléments d'auriculothérapie. Sainte Ruffine: Ed Maisonneuve; 1980
8. Bricot B. Enseignement d'auriculotherapie. Conference, GLEM. Lyon, 1985
9. Egger J. Food allergy and the central nervous system in childhood. In: Brostoff J, Challacombe S. Food allergy and intolerance. London: Baillère Tindal; 1987:pp. 666–673
10. Darlington LG, Ramsey NW. Diets for rheumatoid arthritis. Lancet 1991;338:1209
11. Wraith DG. Asthma. In: Brostoff J, Challacombe S. Food allergy and intolerance. London: Baillère Tindal; 1987:pp. 486–497
12. Alimi D. 5th International Symposium of Auriculomedicine. Conference, GLEM. Lyon, 2006

■ *Further Reading*

Bossy J, Prat-Pradal D, Taillandier J. Les Microsystèmes de l'Acupuncture. Paris: Masson; 1984
Bossy J. Bases Neurobiologiques des Réflexothérapies. Paris: Masson; 1978
Bourdiol RJ. Eléments d'Auriculothérapie. Sainte-Ruffine: Maisonneuve; 1982
Helms JM. Acupuncture Energetics: A Clinical Approach for Physicians. New York: Thieme Medical Publishers; 2008
Leclerc B. Auriculothérapie Théorique et Pratique. Published by the author himself. Nevers; 1996
Nogier PFM. Traité d'Auriculothérapie. Sainte-Ruffine: Maisonneuve; 1969
Nogier PFM, Nogier R. The Man in the Ear. Sainte-Ruffine: Maisonneuve; 1985
Nogier PFM. Introduction Pratique a l'Auriculothérapie. Brussels: SATAS; 1999
Nogier PFM, Maillard A, Petitjean F, Grignard Ph. Points Réflexes Auriculaires. Sainte-Ruffine: Maisonneuve; 1987
Nogier PFM, Petitjean F, Maillard A. Compléments des Points Réflexes Auriculaires. Sainte-Ruffine: Maisonneuve; 1989

Nogier PFM. From Auriculotherapy to Auricular Medicine. Sainte-Ruffine, France: Maisonneuve; 1983

Oleson TD. Auriculotherapy Manual: Chinese and Western Systems of Ear Acupuncture, 2nd ed. Los Angeles: Health Care Alternatives; 1996

Rouxeville Y. Abrégé de cours d'Auriculothérapie et d'Auriculomédicine. Published by the author himself (out of stock); 1993

Rouxeville Y. Acupuncture Auriculaire Personnalisée. Montpellier: Sauramps Médical; 2000

Index

Please note: page numbers in *italics* refer to figures on that page.